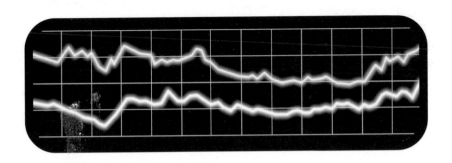

NORMAL VALUES IN PREGNANCY

D1428414

Commissioning Editor **Miranda Bromage**
Production Manager **Mark Sanderson**
Design Direction **Deborah Gyan**

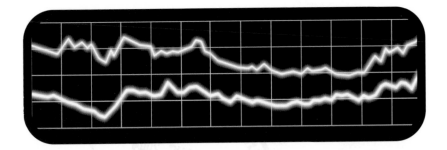

NORMAL VALUES IN PREGNANCY

MM RAMSAY MA, MD, MRCOG, MRCP
Senior Lecturer in Fetomaternal Medicine
Academic Division of Obstetrics and Gynaecology
School of Human Development, University of Nottingham
Queen's Medical Centre Nottingham, UK

DK JAMES MA, MD, FRCOG, DCH
Professor of Fetomaternal Medicine
Academic Division of Obstetrics and Gynaecology
School of Human Development, University of Nottingham
Queen's Medical Centre Nottingham, UK

PJ STEER BSc, MD, FRCOG
Professor, Academic Department of Obstetrics and Gynaecology
Charing Cross and Westminster Medical School
Chelsea and Westminster Hospital, London, UK

CP WEINER MD
Professor and Chairman, Department of Obstetrics, Gynecology and
Reproductive Sciences
University of Maryland School of Medicine
Baltimore, Maryland, USA

B GONIK MD
Professor and Vice Chairman
Department of Obstetrics and Gynecology
Wayne State University School of Medicine
Grace Hospital, Detroit, Michigan, USA

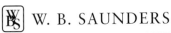 W. B. SAUNDERS

London • Edinburgh • New York • Philadelphia • St Louis • Sydney • Toronto 2000

WB SAUNDERS

An imprint of Harcourt Publishers Limited

First published 2000

ISBN 0-7020-2527-5   √6r0

British Library Cataloging in Publication Data
A catalogue record for this book is available from the British Library

Library of Congress Cataloging in Publication Data
A catalog record for this book is available from the Library of Congress

Note
Medical knowledge is constantly changing. As new information becomes available, changes in treatment, procedures, equipment and the use of drugs become necessary. The editors/authors/contributors and the publishers have taken care to ensure that the information given in this text is accurate and up to date. However, readers are strongly advised to confirm that the information, especially with regard to drug usage, complies with the latest legislation and standards of practice.

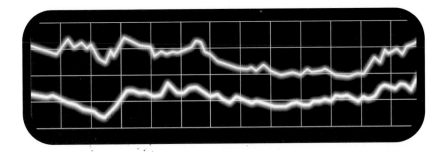

CONTENTS

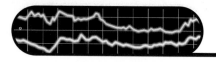

CONTENTS

CONTENTS

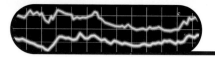

CONTENTS

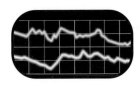

INTRODUCTION

What is a 'normal' value?

'Normal' has different meanings. In the context of physical or laboratory measurements, 'normal' may mean 'average', 'disease-free', or 'within a given statistical range'. However, it is important to know the characteristics of the population yielding 'normal' values before deciding whether they form an appropriate reference range with respect to an individual under study. Many laboratories now print reference ranges on their reports and highlight test values that fall outside these values as 'abnormal'. Where the test subject is a pregnant woman, fetus in utero or a newborn baby and the reference population is comprised predominantly of middle-aged men, then the comparisons are patently inappropriate. It is important first to understand how the physiological changes of pregnancy affect the results of various tests and measurements before deciding whether an out-of-range result is actually abnormal.

Changes in pregnancy

Pregnancy results in profound changes in maternal physiology and metabolism, orchestrated by hormonal changes. Thus, physical and laboratory measurements may be very different in the pregnant as compared to the non-pregnant state, and may also change as pregnancy advances. Similarly, physical, biochemical, hormonal, and hematological measurements of the fetus change markedly as the fetus grows in size and maturity. The fetus, once hidden within the uterus, is now accessible, thanks to ultrasound techniques. Fetal structures can be measured, fetal behavior observed, blood velocities measured with Doppler ultrasound, and the sampling needle can access blood, liquor, urine, and placental and other tissues.

Statistical terms

The terms used to define 'normal' values depend on the distribution characteristics of data points. The entire range of values encountered in a healthy population may be quoted as reference points, or distribution may be described by terms expressing central tendency and scatter. Where data are symmetrically distributed around a central value (i.e. a normal distribution), then mean, standard deviation, and standard error of the mean are the appropriate statistics. From these, ranking values or centiles may be calculated, e.g. 5th and 95th centiles which encompass the central 90% of data points, with 5% either side of them. Where the data distribution is skewed, then median and centiles should be used. With an exponential distribution of data points, then median and multiples of the median can be used rather than centiles. Readers are referred to specialized texts for more detailed critical appraisal of the statistical analyses used in the studies described here (Altman 1991).

Methodology of studies used to derive 'normal' values during pregnancy

There are two basic designs for studies addressing changes in physical or laboratory values during pregnancy:

(i) Longitudinal studies follow a group of women sequentially through pregnancy and compare measurements of a particular parameter with those obtained well before or at an interval after the pregnancy. As these studies are very labor-intensive and require committed research subjects, they tend not to involve very large numbers of subjects. They are very good at demonstrating changes with time, either between non-pregnant and pregnant states or with advancing gestation. The variability of the data is small because the same subjects are studied sequentially. They are very helpful in showing how pregnancy affects measurement of a particular parameter. This has particular relevance when considering a test result for a patient, where values are known pre-pregnancy and the impact of the pregnant state needs to be separated from changes with time due to a disease state. A limitation of longitudinal studies, however, is that a narrow range of 'normal' values is defined from the small numbers of subjects, which does not correspond to the wider range of values found in a larger group of healthy subjects studied on a single occasion.

(ii) Cross-sectional studies involve large numbers of subjects, each contributing one data point to the study. If the numbers included in the study are large enough, then a good idea of the true scatter of data points is obtained. These allow accurate characterisation of mean values, standard deviations and centiles. For pregnancy studies, it is important to have subjects evenly distributed throughout gestation and not to extrapolate values beyond the gestational range actually included. Such studies are essential when it is important to determine the ranking of a particular measurement, e.g. a fetal ultrasonic measurement of abdominal circumference, as on the 10th centile for a known gestational age. Most studies of fetal ultrasonic measurements and Doppler waveform indices are of this design, and their statistical methodology has been described in detail (Altman and Chitty 1994).

There are also opportunistic studies, for example in the fetus, when blood sampling has been done to investigate infection or karyotype, but the fetus found not to be affected by the condition. Any of the blood sample not used for specific tests has then been used to measure other substances. Much of the information available about fetal hematological, biochemical, and endocrine function has been collected in this way. There are obvious ethical difficulties of planning studies in absolutely 'normal' fetuses requiring invasive sampling, as there are risks of fetal injury and loss. However, the selection of fetuses for study following exclusion of a particular problem means that they are not truly 'normal' or representative of the entire fetal population. Opportunistic studies do not cover the entire range of gestational ages. Nevertheless, they provide information that would otherwise not be known.

The pregnancy studies published in the literature are of mixed quality in terms of numbers of subjects included, selection criteria for subjects, sampling and laboratory techniques, and statistical interpretation. We report the best studies found. The methodology for each study included in this book has been described briefly and presented alongside the results. Comment sections provide some interpretation of the data or the robustness of the statistical methods; references to the original papers are given for readers who wish to explore in greater detail. Very few studies address the

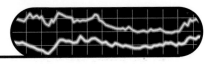

possible influence of maternal age, gravidity, or ethnic differences on the parameters under study. Data on many normal ranges are deficient or limited, and occasionally unreliable. We would welcome new information to fill in these gaps in future editions of this book. All such contributions would be fully acknowledged.

Use of normal ranges in pregnancy

Some disease states are diagnosed from characteristic symptoms or signs, but others have agreed biochemical definitions. For example, diabetes mellitus is diagnosed with reference to fasting blood glucose measurements and those after a known glucose challenge (see Fig. 24). These values represent the upper limits of the 'normal ranges' found in studies of healthy subjects. The pregnancy differences in blood glucose values have led to the suggestion that diagnostic criteria for diabetes should be adjusted in pregnancy.

Disease or organ dysfunction does not always occur at a given value of a physical or laboratory measurement outside its derived normal range. Elevated liver enzymes indicative of liver cell dysfunction may be 2, 10, or 50 times normal values. However, even minimal deviation of pH from its closely clustered normal values may be biologically very important.

Another use of 'normal values' is in the calculation of odds ratios. Assessment of the risk or likelihood of genetic abnormalities (e.g. Down's syndrome) is possible from measurement of serum α-fetoprotein, chorionic gonadotropin or placental protein-A levels (see Fig 44–46). Measured values of these hormones are compared with expected values at known gestational age (derived from healthy pregnancies). The degree of difference is expressed in terms of multiples of the median (MoM) values. Absolute values cannot be used for mathematical calculations as these hormonal concentrations change with gestation. For each hormone, multiple regression analysis has shown the relationships between deviations in its values and risk of Down's syndrome. Thus, a woman's age-related risk of aneuploidy may be adjusted following measurement of serum hormones (Wald et al, 1996).

Units of measurement

Where possible, both SI and traditional units have been given for ease of interpretation. It is important to check the units of measurement carefully when comparing a physical or laboratory value with a 'normal range'. In SI units, grams (g) and liters (L) are used, whereas traditional units commonly employ milligrams (mg) and deciliters (dl). The prefixes d, m, μ, and n, signifying 10^{-1}, 10^{-3}, 10^{-6}, and 10^{-9}, must be observed and used with care, in order to avoid errors of interpretation.

The terminology 'milliequivalents' (mEq) has not been used, as it has been superceded by millimoles (mmol). Readers are reminded that for monovalent ions (Na+, K+, Cl−) 1 mmol = 1 mEq. For divalent ions (Mg^{2+}, Ca^{2+}, PO_4^{2+}, SO_4^{2-}) 1 mmol = 2 mEq.

Conclusion

We believe this book will educate regarding many aspects of maternal and fetal physiology as well as be an invaluable reference text for all practising obstetricians, internists, general practitioners, midwives, and nurses dealing with women in pregnancy. The book will also be extremely useful to undergraduate and postgraduate students in obstetrics and perinatal medicine.

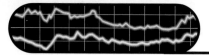

Further reading

Altman DG (1991) Practical statistics for medical research. Chapman and Hall, London.

Altman DG, Chitty LS (1994) Charts of fetal size: 1. Methodology. Br J Obstet Gynecol 101: 29–34.

Wald NJ, George L, Smith D, Densem JW, Petterson K (1996) Serum screening for Down's syndrome between 8 and 14 weeks of pregnancy. Br J Obstet Gynaecol 103: 407–412.

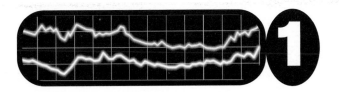

MATERNAL VALUES

PHYSIOLOGY
BIOCHEMISTRY
HEMATOLOGY
IMMUNOLOGY
ENDOCRINOLOGY

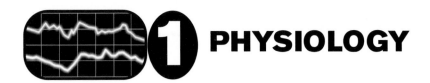

PHYSIOLOGY

NUTRITION

Weight gain

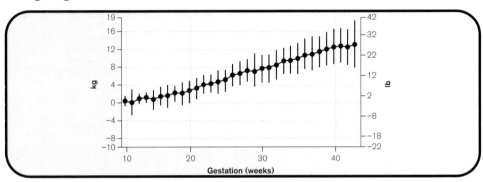

Figure 1 Maternal weight gain (mean ± SD) in 988 normal women who had uneventful pregnancies; all booked at <20 weeks and delivered between 37 and 41 weeks' gestation. (Longitudinal study.) *Data source*: ref. 1, with permission.

Weight-for-height category	Recommended total weight gain	
	kg	lb
Low (BMI <19.8)	12.5–18	28–40
Normal (BMI 19.8–26.0)	11.5–16	25–35
High (BMI 26.0–29.0)	7–11.5	15–25
Obese (BMI >29.0)	7	15
BMI = weight/height^2)		

Figure 2 Recommended total body weight gain ranges for women during pregnancy with a singleton gestation, classified by pre-pregnancy body mass index (BMI). *Data source*: ref. 2, with permission, National Academy Press.

Comment: Average total weight gain during pregnancy is approximately 10 kg. Low weight gain during pregnancy in non-obese women has been associated with delivery of small-for-gestational-age infants.[3] However, overweight women often deliver large-for-gestational-age infants, regardless of their weight gain during pregnancy.[3]

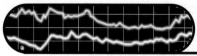

Nutritional requirements

Nutrient (unit)	Pregnant	Lactating
Energy (kcal)	+300	+500
Protein (g)	60	65
Fat-soluable vitamins		
Vitamin A (μg retinol equivalents)	800	1300
Vitamin D (μg as cholecalciferol)	10	10
Vitamin E (mg α-tocopherol equivalents)	10	12
Vitamin K (μg)	65	65
Water-soluble vitamins		
Vitamin C (mg)	70	95
Thiamin (mg)	1.5	1.6
Riboflavin (mg)	1.6	1.8
Niacin (mg niacin equivalent)	17	20
Vitamin B_6 (mg)	2.2	2.1
Folate (μg)	400	280
Vitamin B_{12} (μg)	2.2	2.6
Minerals		
Calcium (mg)	1200	1200
Phosphorus (mg)	1200	1200
Magnesium (mg)	300	355
Iron (mg)	30	15
Zinc (mg)	15	19
Iodine (μg)	175	200
Selenium (μg)	65	75

Figure 3 Recommended daily dietary allowances and energy intakes for women while pregnant and lactating. These should be used as a guide to nutritional requirements when formulating a balanced diet. *Data source*: ref. 4, with permission, National Academy Press.

Comment: The increased requirements during pregnancy for vitamins and minerals can usually be met from the diet, thus routine supplementation with multivitamin preparations is not necessary. However, periconceptual supplementation with folic acid for all women in pregnancy is now advocated in an attempt to reduce the incidence of neural tube defects. Vitamin supplementation should be considered in women with inadequate standard diets, heavy smokers, drug or alcohol abusers, or those with multiple pregnancies. Excessive intake (i.e. more than twice the recommended daily allowance) of vitamins (fat- or water-soluble) may have toxic effects.

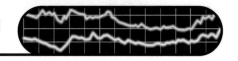

CARDIOVASCULAR FUNCTION

Blood pressure

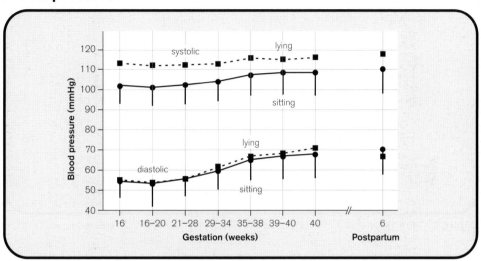

Figure 4 Blood pressure measurements (mean and standard deviation (SD)) from a longitudinal study of 226 primigravidae whose first attendance at the antenatal clinic was before 20 weeks of pregnancy. Their mean age was 24.3 years (SD 4.9 years). Blood pressure measurements were taken with the London School of Hygiene sphygmomanometer to avoid terminal digit preference and observer bias; diastolic pressures were recorded at the point of muffling (phase 4). *Data source*: ref. 5, with permission, Portland Press Limited.

Comment: Systolic pressure changes little during pregnancy, but diastolic pressure falls markedly toward mid-pregnancy, then rising to near non-pregnant levels by term. Thus, there is a widening of the pulse pressure for most of the pregnancy.

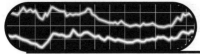

Pulse rate

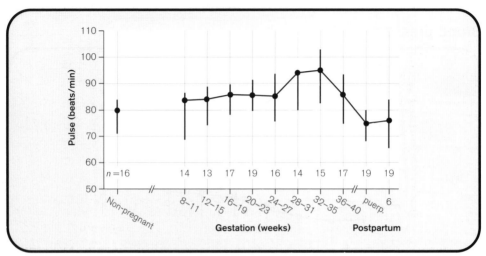

Figure 5 Pulse rate (median and interquartile (IQ) ranges) from a longitudinal study of 20 healthy women recruited in early pregnancy and studied every 2 weeks thereafter; 'non-pregnant' measurements were made 8–12 months after delivery. All women finished the study but not all participated in every visit. *Data source:* ref. 6, with permission.

Comment: The typical increase in heart rate during pregnancy is approximately 15 beats/min, present from as early as 4 weeks after the last menstrual period.[7]

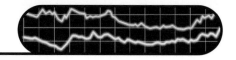

Cardiac output

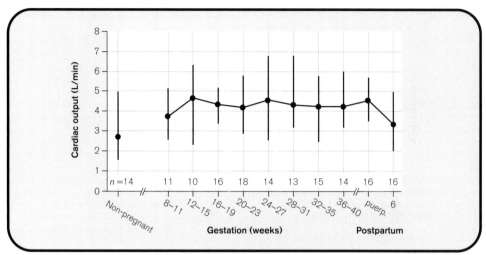

Figure 6 Cardiac output (median and IQ ranges) from a longitudinal study of 20 healthy women recruited in early pregnancy and studied every 2 weeks thereafter; 'non-pregnant' measurements were made 8–12 months after delivery. All women finished the study but not all participated in every visit. Cardiac output was measured by an indirect Fick method. *Data source*: ref. 6, with permission.

Comment: Cardiac output increases significantly during the first trimester and thereafter remains elevated until the puerperium. When changes in body weight are taken into consideration, it is apparent that cardiac output reaches maximal values between 12 and 15 weeks' gestation and thereafter declines gradually towards term.

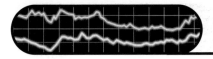

Invasive monitoring

	Non-pregnant	Pregnant
Cardiac output (L/min)	4.3 ± 0.9	6.2 ± 1.0
Heart rate (beats/min)	71 ± 10	83 ± 10
Systemic vascular resistance (dyne s cm^{-5})	1530 ± 520	1210 ± 266
Pulmonary vascular resistance (dyne s cm^{-5})	119 ± 47	78 ± 22
Colloid oncotic pressure (mmHg)	20.8 ± 1.0	18.0 ± 1.5
Colloid oncotic pressure – pulmonary capillary wedge pressure (mmHg)	14.5 ± 2.5	10.5 ± 2.7
Mean arterial pressure (mmHg)	86.4 ± 7.5	90.3 ± 5.8
Pulmonary capillary wedge pressure (mmHg)	6.3 ± 2.1	7.5 ± 1.8
Central venous pressure (mmHg)	3.7 ± 2.6	3.6 ± 2.5
Left ventricular stroke work index (g min m^{-2})	41 ± 8	48 ± 6

Figure 7 Study involving 10 healthy, primigravid women with a singleton pregnancy examined between 36 and 38 weeks' gestation and then again between 11 and 13 weeks' postpartum. All women were less than 26 years old, non-smokers, and not anemic, and there was normal fetal anatomy, growth, and amniotic fluid volume. A pulmonary artery catheter was placed via the subclavian vein, and baseline hemodynamic assessment was made in the left lateral position after 30 min of rest. Cardiac output was measured with a thermodilution technique (and for each subject the result represented the mean of five independent measurements with the highest and lowest values excluded); central pressures were measured over three consecutive respiratory cycles. Results quoted are means ± SD. *Data source*: ref. 8, with permission.

Comment: Systemic vascular resistance is 21% lower and pulmonary resistance is 34% lower in the late third trimester than in the non-pregnant state. Both colloid oncotic pressure and the colloid oncotic–pulmonary capillary wedge pressure gradient are also lower (by 14 and 28%, respectively). There are no significant changes in the third trimester with respect to mean arterial pressure, central venous pressure, pulmonary capillary wedge pressure, or left ventricular stroke work index. These results indicate that both systemic and pulmonary vascular beds accommodate higher vascular volumes at normal pressures during pregnancy, the ventricles are dilated, and cardiac contractility does not change significantly. Since the colloid oncotic pressure–pulmonary capillary wedge pressure gradient is reduced in pregnancy, any increase in cardiac preload or any alteration in pulmonary capillary permeability will predispose to pulmonary edema.

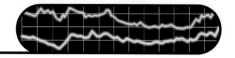

PULMONARY FUNCTION AND RESPIRATION

Arterial blood gases

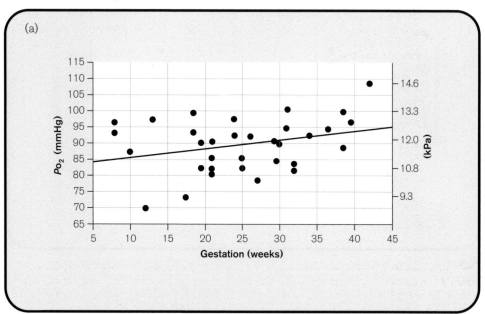

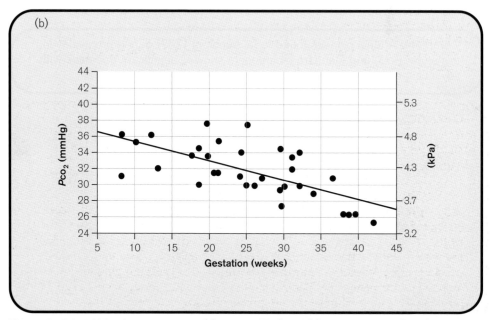

Figure 8 Arterial blood gas pressures: (a) oxygen (P_{O_2}) and (b) carbon dioxide (P_{CO_2}).

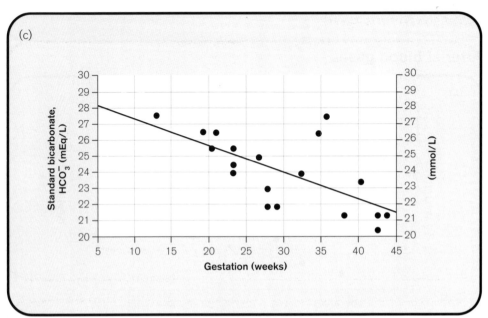

Figure 8 Arterial blood gas pressures: (c) standard bicarbonate (individual values, with regression lines shown) from a cross-sectional study of 37 women between 8 and 42 weeks of pregnancy. Blood sampling was done from a cannula inserted into the brachial artery under local anesthesia, after 30 min of rest in a quiet, darkened room. *Data source:* ref. 9, with permission from Elsevier Science.

Comment: Arterial pH was found to be constant (7.47) during pregnancy in this study. P_{CO_2} and standard bicarbonate showed significant decrease with advancing gestation, but P_{O_2} levels did not alter significantly.

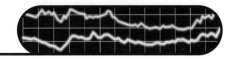

Transcutaneous gases

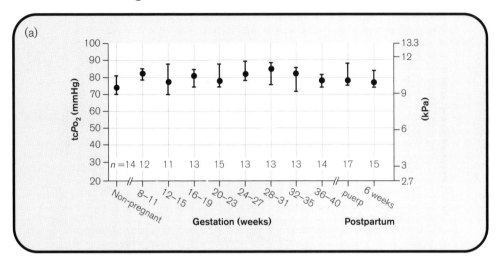

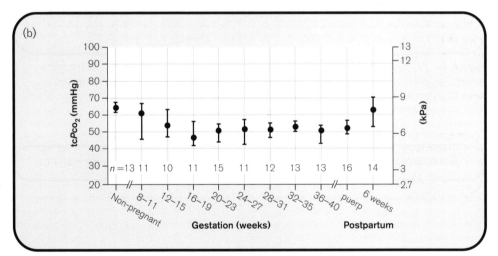

Figure 9 (a) Transcutaneous oxygen (tcP_{O_2}) and (b) carbon dioxide (tcP_{CO_2}) pressures (median and IQ ranges) from a longitudinal study of 20 healthy women recruited in early pregnancy and studied every 2 weeks thereafter; 'non-pregnant' measurements were made 8–12 months after delivery. All women finished the study but not all participated in every visit. *Data source:* ref. 6, with permission.

Comment: Transcutaneous P_{CO_2} is higher than arterial P_{CO_2} due to temperature differences between the skin surface and blood, as well as addition of CO_2 by skin metabolism (conversion factor *approximately* 1.4).[6] Transcutaneous P_{O_2} values in adults are 10–20% lower than arterial P_{O_2} values. In this study the rise in tcP_{O_2} and fall in tcP_{CO_2} during pregnancy were both significant.

Respiration rate

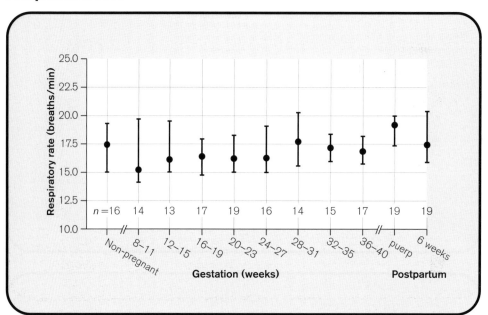

Figure 10 Respiration rate (median and IQ ranges) from a longitudinal study of 20 healthy women recruited in early pregnancy and studied every 2 weeks thereafter; 'non-pregnant' measurements were made 8–12 months after delivery. All women finished the study but not all participated in every visit. *Data source*: ref. 6, with permission.

Comment: Respiration rate is similar in pregnant and non-pregnant women.

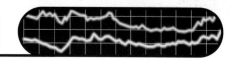

Tidal volume

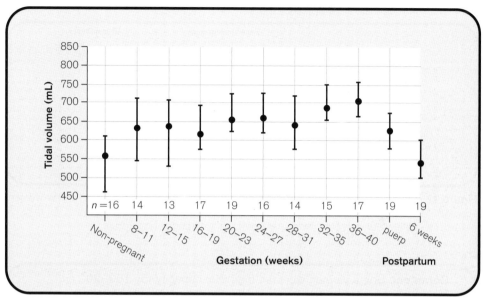

Figure 11 Tidal volume (medium and IQ ranges) from a longitudinal study of 20 healthy women recruited in early pregnancy and studied every 2 weeks thereafter; 'non-pregnant' measurements were made 8–12 months after delivery. All women finished the study but not all participated in every visit. *Data source*: ref. 6, with permission.

Comment: Tidal volume increases early in pregnancy and continues to rise until term; overall, there is a 30–40% rise. By 6–8 weeks postpartum, tidal volumes have returned to non-pregnant values. Minute ventilation rises in parallel with tidal volume; typical values are 7.5 L/min for a non-pregnant woman, and 10.5 L/min in late pregnancy.[10]

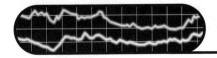

Respiratory function tests

	During pregnancy			After delivery
	10 weeks	24 weeks	36 weeks	10 weeks postpartum
Vital capacity (L)	3.8	3.9	4.1	3.8
Inspiratory capacity (L)	2.6	2.7	2.9	2.5
Expiratory reserve volume (L)	1.2	1.2	1.2	1.3
Residual volume (L)	1.2	1.1	1.0	1.2

Figure 12 Respiratory volumes (mean values) from a longitudinal study of eight healthy women, aged 18–29 years, studied through pregnancy and then again 10 weeks postpartum. All tests were done in the sitting position. *Data source*: ref. 10, with permission.

Comment: Some women increase their vital capacity (by 100–200 mL) during pregnancy, but the converse has been demonstrated in obese women.[11] Anatomical changes (flaring of the lower ribs, a rise in the diaphragm, and increase in transverse diameter of the chest) are responsible for the alterations in lung volume subdivisions.[11] Forced expiratory volume in 1 s (FEV_1) and peak expiratory flow rate (PEFR) are unaffected by normal pregnancy.[10] The gas transfer factor (i.e. pulmonary diffusing capacity with carbon monoxide) decreases in pregnancy.[10] This has been attributed to altered mucopolysaccharides in the alveolar capillary walls, as well as a lower circulating hemoglobin level.

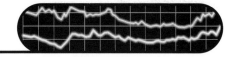

CHROMOSOMAL ABNORMALITIES

Maternal age at delivery (years)	Risk of Down's syndrome
15	1 : 1578
20	1 : 1528
25	1 : 1351
30	1 : 909
31	1 : 796
32	1 : 683
33	1 : 574
34	1 : 474
35	1 : 384
36	1 : 307
37	1 : 242
38	1 : 189
39	1 : 146
40	1 : 112
41	1 : 85
42	1 : 65
43	1 : 49
44	1 : 37
45	1 : 28
46	1 : 21
47	1 : 15
48	1 : 11
49	1 : 8
50	1 : 6

Figure 13 Risk of having a pregnancy associated with Down's syndrome according to maternal age at time of birth. *Data source*: ref. 12, with permission.

Maternal age	Rate per 1000				
	Trisomy 21	Trisomy 18	Trisomy 13	XXY	All chromosomal anomalies
35	3.9	0.5	0.2	0.5	8.7
36	5.0	0.7	0.3	0.6	10.1
37	6.4	1.0	0.4	0.8	12.2
38	8.1	1.4	0.5	1.1	14.8
39	10.4	2.0	0.8	1.4	18.4
40	13.3	2.8	1.1	1.8	23.0
41	16.9	3.9	1.5	2.4	29.0
42	21.6	5.5	2.1	3.1	37.0
43	27.4	7.6		4.1	45.0
44	34.8			5.4	50.0
45	44.2			7.0	62.0
46	55.9			9.1	77.0
47	70.4			11.9	96.0

Figure 14 Chromosomal abnormalities by maternal age at time of amniocentesis at 16 weeks' gestation (expressed as rate per 1000). *Data source*: ref. 13, with permission.

Comment: The incidence of chromosomal disorders rises with increasing maternal age, but is not influenced by paternal age.[13] Trisomy 21 (Down's syndrome) is the most important numerically of these disorders, with an overall population incidence of 1 in 650 live births. Trisomies 13, 18, and 22 are rare as live births. Other autosomal trisomies are non-viable and are commonly found in spontaneous abortions.

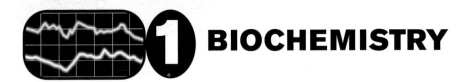

1 BIOCHEMISTRY

Total serum protein and albumin

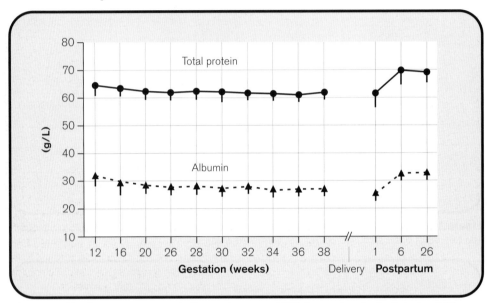

Figure 15 Total serum protein and albumin (mean and SD) from a longitudinal study of 83 healthy pregnant women (77 of whom were primigravidae), recruited at 12 weeks' gestation. Samples were collected every 4 weeks during pregnancy, 7 days postpartum, then at 6 and 26 weeks postpartum. *Data source*: ref. 14, with permission.

Comment: Decreased total serum protein and albumin concentrations in pregnancy are associated with a decrease in colloid osmotic pressure.[14] Serum immunoglobulin levels do not change significantly in pregnancy.[15]

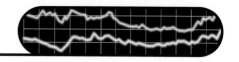

Liver enzymes, serum bile acids, bilirubin, amylase, copper and zinc

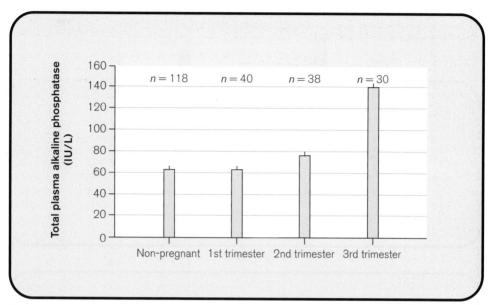

Figure 16 Total alkaline phosphatase levels (mean and standard error of the mean (SEM)) from a cross-sectional study of 108 normal women attending a hospital antenatal clinic in Nigeria; the non-pregnant controls of similar age were patients attending the gynecological clinic. No patients were clinically anemic and all were normotensive. *Data source*: ref. 16, with permission.

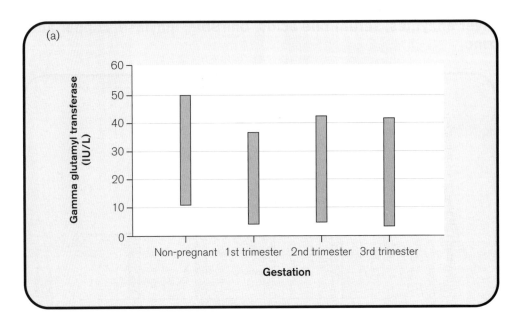

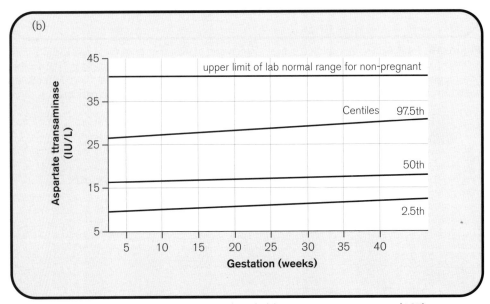

Figure 17 (a) Serum γ-glutamyl transferase (GGT), (b) aspartate transaminase (AST).

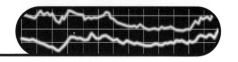

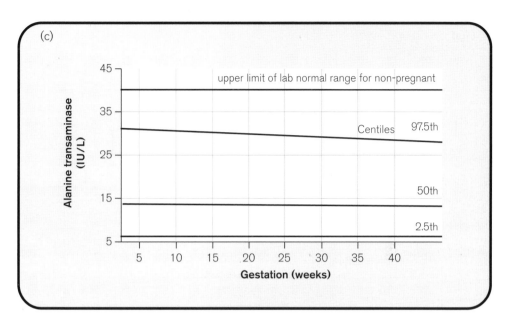

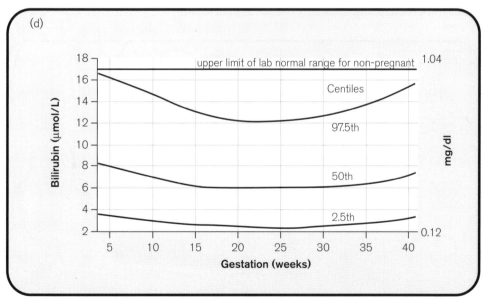

Figure 17 (c) alanine transaminase (ALT), (d) bilirubin levels (95% reference ranges) from a cross-sectional study of 430 women with uncomplicated singleton pregnancy. All subjects were free from hypertension or liver disease and none was taking drugs associated with liver dysfunction or consuming more than 10 units of alcohol per week. Data for GGT were not normally distributed, and the results presented are calculated from the non-parametric determination of percentiles. Data for AST, ALT, and bilirubin were normally distributed after logarithmic transformation, allowing gestation-specific centiles to be calculated. *Data source*: ref. 17, with permission.

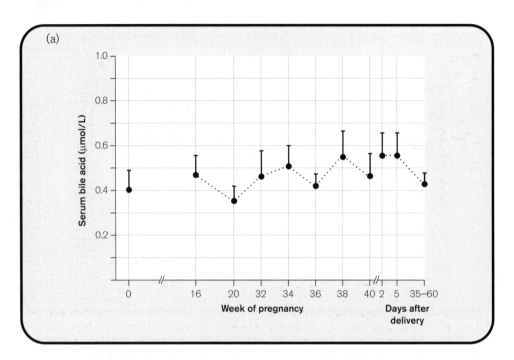

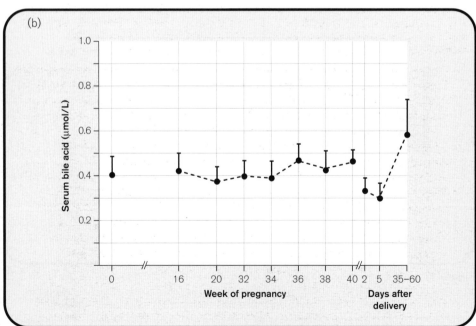

Figure 18 (a) Serum cholic acid (CA), (b) deoxycholic acid (DCA).

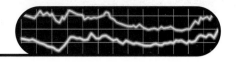

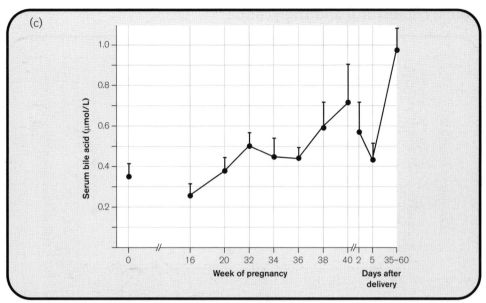

Figure 18 (c) chemodeoxycholic acid (CDCA) levels (mean and SD) from a longitudinal study of 30 healthy pregnant women. They had no history of hepatobiliary disease, and their pregnancies were uncomplicated. Blood samples were taken after overnight fasting. Most women were recruited at 12–17 weeks' gestation and they continued giving blood samples at 18–22 weeks, every 2 weeks in the third trimester and until 35–60 days post-delivery. Bile acids were measured separately by radioimmunoassays, and the results presented are for total concentrations (i.e. free plus conjugated bile acid). *Data source*: ref. 18, with permission.

Comment: Total plasma alkaline phosphatase (AP) levels are approximately doubled by late pregnancy. Almost half of the total plasma AP in pregnancy is placental AP isoenzyme, but bone AP isoenzyme levels are also markedly increased; liver AP isoenzyme levels do not change significantly in pregnancy.[16] Serum GGT and transaminase levels overall are lower in pregnancy than in the non-pregnant adult population. There are no significant gestational changes in GGT, AST, or ALT, or during labor or the puerperium.[19] Bilirubin levels remain within normal adult levels during pregnancy.[20] The primary bile acid, CA, and the secondary bile acid, DCA, do not change in serum concentrations during pregnancy, but CDCA levels rise significantly towards term.[18] These minor changes in serum bile acids may be due to changes in bile acid metabolism and excretion brought about by high circulating estrogen and progesterone levels, but could indicate a tendency to cholestasis in normal pregnancy. No data are available regarding serum amylase in pregnancy, but decreased concentrations may be expected as a dilutional effect. Serum copper levels are increased in pregnancy, but zinc levels decreased from those in non-pregnant women.[21] There are considerable differences between laboratories with regard to liver enzyme assays and hence 'normal ranges' in the adult population; these should be borne in mind when interpreting individual results from pregnant women.

Lipids: cholesterol and triglyceride

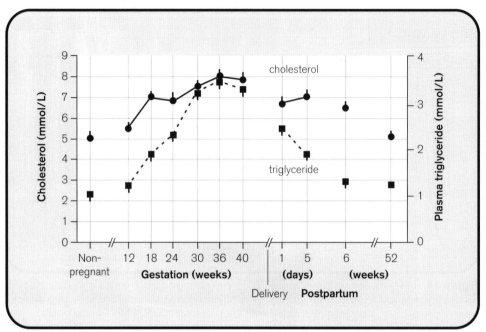

Figure 19 Plasma cholesterol and triglyceride levels (mean and SEM) from a longitudinal study of 43 women aged 20–41 years. Samples were taken following an overnight fast and 10 min of supine rest at 4–6 weekly intervals through pregnancy, during labor, and in the puerperium; and also 12 months after delivery in 14 of the subjects. The non-pregnant reference samples were from 15 subjects of comparable age. No dietary restrictions were imposed. *Data source*: ref. 22, with permission. Conversion factors: cholesterol, mmol/L × 38.5 = mg/dl; triglyceride, mmol/L × 88 = mg/dl

Comment: The plasma cholesterol level doubles and there is a threefold increase in plasma triglyceride concentration during pregnancy. The lipid content of the low-density lipoproteins increases in pregnancy, as does high-density lipoprotein triglyceride content.[22] Serum lipid levels fall rapidly after delivery, but both cholesterol and triglyceride concentrations remain elevated at 6–7 weeks postpartum. Lactation does not influence lipid levels.[22]

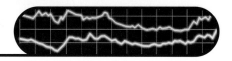

RENAL FUNCTION

Serum urate

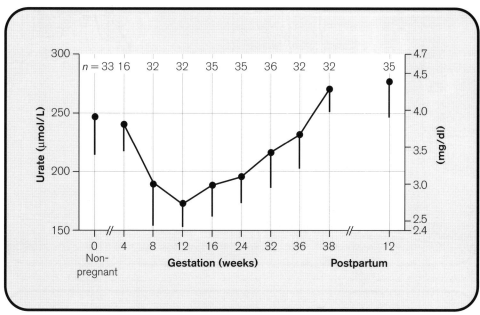

Figure 20 Serum urate levels (mean and SD) from a longitudinal study of 31 healthy women, aged 23–37 years, five of whom were studied during two pregnancies. They were studied preconceptually, at least 3 months after stopping oral contraceptives (if used), in the luteal phase of their menstrual cycle, then monthly during pregnancy and again 12 weeks postpartum. All samples were taken between 0900 and 0930 h, after overnight fasting. *Data source*: ref. 23, with permission.

Comment: Serum urate levels decrease during the first trimester, probably due to altered renal handling of uric acid.[23] During late pregnancy, serum urate rises to reach levels higher than non-pregnant values at term; these may remain elevated for 12 weeks after delivery.[23]

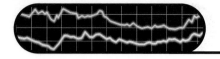

BIOCHEMISTRY

Serum osmolality, electrolytes, and urea

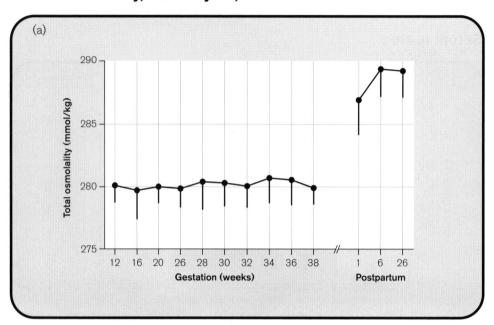

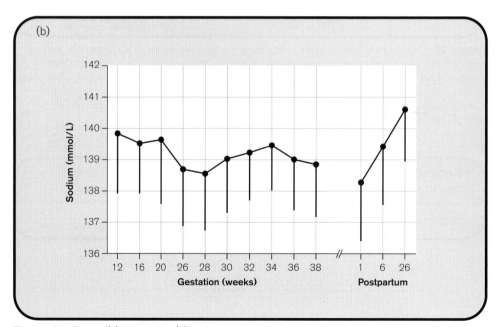

Figure 21 Serum (a) osmolality, (b) sodium.

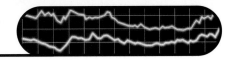

(c)

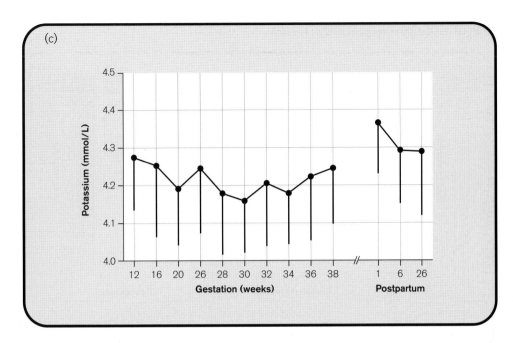

(d)

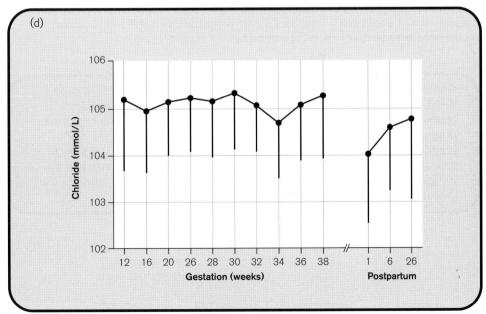

Figure 21 Serum (c) potassium, (d) chloride.

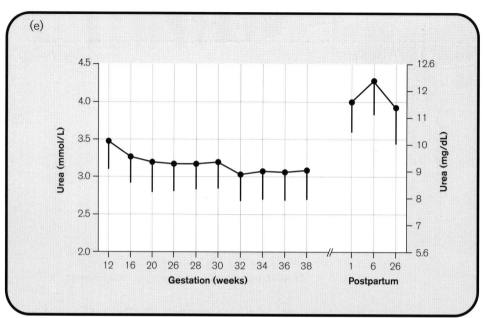

Figure 21 Serum (e) urea (mean and SD) from a longitudinal study of 83 healthy pregnant women (77 of whom were primigravidae), recruited at 12 weeks' gestation. Samples were collected every 4 weeks during pregnancy, 7 days postpartum, then at 6 and 26 weeks postpartum. *Data source*: ref. 14, with permission.

Comment: Total osmolality falls by the end of the first trimester to a nadir 8–10 mmol/kg below non-pregnant values. The major serum electrolytes (sodium, potassium, chloride) have almost unchanged concentrations during pregnancy. Bicarbonate and phosphate concentrations decline during pregnancy.[24] Both plasma urea and creatinine levels fall during pregnancy; typical mean (SD) values for plasma creatinine are 60 (8), 54 (10), and 64 (9) μmol/L in the first, second, and third trimesters respectively, rising to 73 (10) μmol/L by 6 weeks postpartum[25,26] (see also Fig. 22c).

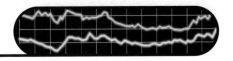

Creatinine clearance and serum creatinine

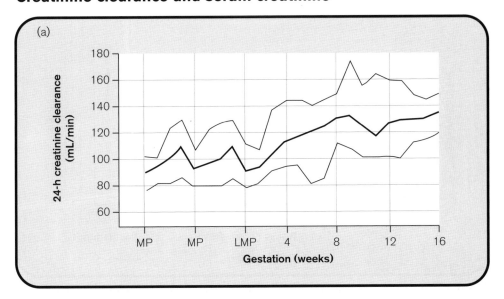

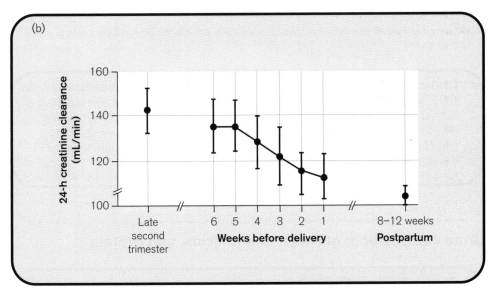

Figure 22 (a) Creatinine clearance (mean and range) in early pregnancy from a longitudinal study of nine healthy women, recruited prior to pregnancy. Measurements of 24 h creatinine clearance were made weekly, through the different phases of the menstrual cycle and up to 16 weeks' gestation. No diet, fluid, or exercise restrictions were imposed. *Data source*: ref. 27, with permission. (b) Creatinine clearance (mean ± SEM) in the second and third trimesters from a longitudinal study of 10 healthy pregnant women. Creatinine clearance measurements were made once between 25 and 28 weeks' gestation, then weekly from 32 weeks until delivery, and finally once between 8 and 12 weeks postpartum. *Data source*: ref. 28, with permission.

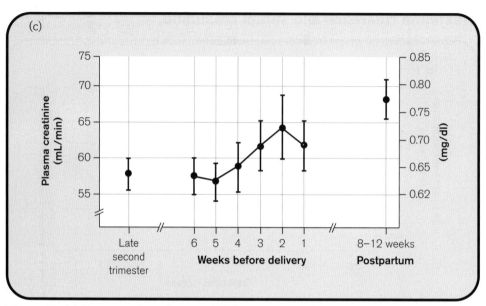

Figure 22 (c) Serum creatinine (mean ± SEM) in the second and third trimesters from a longitudinal study of 10 healthy pregnant women. Creatinine clearance measurements were made once between 25 and 28 weeks' gestation, then weekly from 32 weeks until delivery, and finally once between 8 and 12 weeks postpartum. *Data source:* ref. 28, with permission.

Comment: Glomerular filtration rate (GFR) and effective renal plasma flow increase in early pregnancy to levels approximately 50% above non-pregnant values; in the third trimester, GFR declines by about 15%.[28] 24 h creatinine clearance measurements mirror these changes. During the menstrual cycle, there is a 20% mean increase in creatinine clearance between the week of menstruation and the late luteal phase.[27]

Urine composition: glucose, amino acids, and protein

Comment: Glycosuria is common in pregnancy in individuals whose plasma glucose concentrations and glucose tolerance tests are normal. It is thought to arise because of increased glomerular filtration plus decreased tubular resorption of glucose.[29] Aminoaciduria has also been demonstrated during pregnancy,[30] and there is an increase in urinary albumin excretion.[31]

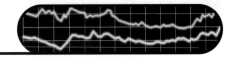

CARBOHYDRATE METABOLISM

Fasting plasma glucose

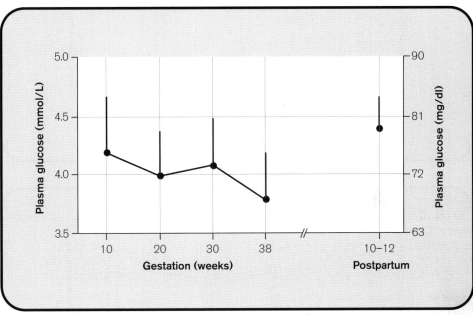

Figure 23 Longitudinal study of plasma glucose levels (mean and SD) following an overnight fast (of at least 10 h duration) in 19 healthy women, none of whom was obese or had a family history of diabetes mellitus. *Data source*: ref. 32, with permission.

Comment: Other studies[33] confirm these findings that fasting plasma glucose levels decrease in pregnancy. In most women that decline has taken place by the end of the first trimester. Thereafter, most studies have documented further decreases in the second and third trimesters.[33] Severely obese women (BMI > 30.0 kg/m²) followed through pregnancy did not show these changes, but rather had progressively rising plasma glucose.[33] Plasma insulin levels rise in the third trimester.[32]

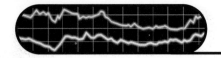
Glucose tolerance test (GTT)

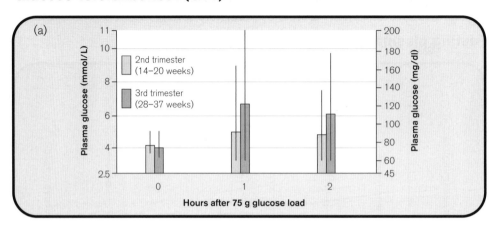

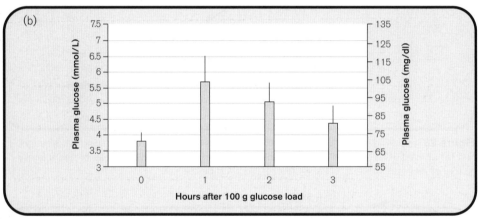

Figure 24 (a) Plasma glucose values (median, 2.5 and 97.5 centiles) after a 75 g oral glucose load. Cross-sectional study of 111 healthy women under the age of 35 years, weighing less than 85.0 kg, with singleton pregnancies ($n = 43$ and 168 in the second and third trimesters, respectively). None had a personal or family history of diabetes mellitus. *Data source:* ref. 34, with permission. (b) Plasma glucose values (mean and SD) after a 100 g oral glucose load. Study involving 752 unselected pregnancies ($n = 20$, 339, and 393 in the first, second, and third trimesters respectively). *Data source:* ref. 35, with permission.

Comment: Women in the third trimester have decreased glucose tolerance, as judged by criteria used to diagnose diabetes outside pregnancy. It has been proposed that gestational diabetes may be diagnosed when two or more of the following plasma glucose levels are found in a 100 g GTT: $\geq$ 105 mg/dL (fasting), $\geq$ 190 mg/dL (1 h), 165 mg/dL (2 h), $\geq$ 145 mg/dL (3 h). These values are 5.8 mmol/L (fasting), 10.6 mmol/L (1 h), 9.2 mmol/L (2 h), 8.1 mmol/L (3 h).[36]

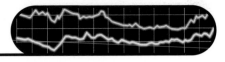

Serum fructosamine and glycosylated hemoglobin

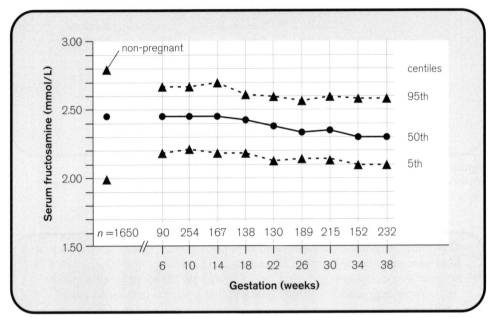

Figure 25 Serum fructosamine levels (median, 5th and 95th centiles) from a cross-sectional study of 1200 pregnant women at different gestational ages, compared to 1650 non-pregnant women, aged between 15 and 40 years. Women with known diabetes or previous gestational diabetes were excluded from the study. *Data source:* ref. 37, with permission.

Comment: Serum fructosamine concentrations are significantly lower in the second and third trimesters than in the first trimester or non-pregnant state. Falling total protein and albumin concentrations in pregnancy may contribute to this reduction in serum fructosamine levels.[37] Values for glycosylated hemoglobin (Hb A_1 and Hb A_{1c}) during pregnancy in healthy women have been shown in some studies to be lower in the first and second trimesters[33,38] but in other studies to be similar to values found in non-pregnant women.[39]

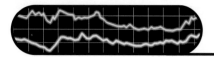

Amniotic fluid insulin, glucose, and C-peptide

		Glucose (mmol/L)	Immunoreactive insulin (pmol/L)	C-peptide (pmol/L)	C-peptide/ insulin molar ratio
Early pregnancy	$n = 77$	3.44 ± 0.22	44.2 ± 2.1	38 ± 2.0	0.97 ± 0.06
Late pregnancy	$n = 33$	0.72 ± 0.11	45.5 ± 2.6	218 ± 54	4.3 ± 1.2

Figure 26 Amniotic fluid insulin, glucose, and C-peptide levels (mean and SD) from a cross-sectional study of 110 non-diabetic women who had amniocentesis performed in pregnancy (mostly for karyotyping). *Data source:* ref. 40, with permission.

Comment: Amniotic fluid insulin and C-peptide can be studied as markers of fetal pancreatic β-cell function. C-peptide and insulin are normally secreted in equimolar amounts from β-cells; C-peptide may be the more reliable marker as insulin is degraded in the fetal liver and there may be circulating insulin antibodies.[40] In diabetic pregnancies, concentrations of these substances are greater, and third trimester values are correlated with neonatal complications (macrosomia, hypoglycemia, jaundice, respiratory distress).[41] The amniotic fluid insulin concentration in the middle trimester has also been shown to be greater in women who subsequently develop gestational diabetes.[42]

ANTIOXIDANTS

Comment: In pregnancy, levels of vitamin E (a free radical scavenger which opposes the effects of lipid peroxides) are increased, compared to the non-pregnant state.[43] Vitamin E levels have been shown to rise progressively with gestation, whereas lipid peroxide levels remain constant.[43] Ascorbic acid concentrations in maternal serum during the third trimester of pregnancy and in breast milk during lactation relate to dietary consumption of fruit and vegetables.[44]

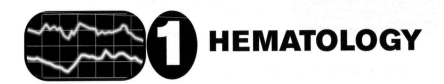

HEMATOLOGY

WHITE CELL COUNT (TOTAL AND DIFFERENTIAL)

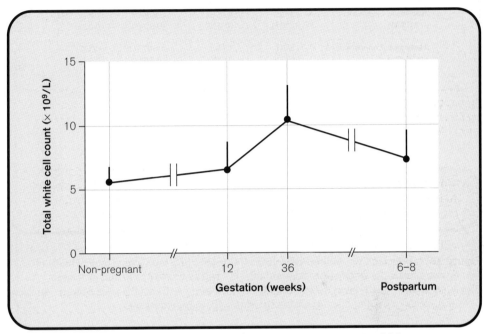

Figure 27 Total white cell count (mean and SD) from a longitudinal study of 24 women recruited at 12 weeks, who delivered after 37 weeks. 'Non-pregnant' samples were taken 4–6 months post-delivery. Samples were analyzed in a Coulter counter. *Data source:* ref. 45, with permission.

Comment: Supplementation with iron and folate does not affect the total white cell count during or after pregnancy. Pregnancy-related changes in the white cell count are still present 6–8 weeks post-delivery. Another (cross-sectional) study found no change in numbers of circulating lymphocytes and monocytes, but decreased eosinophils in the third trimester.[46] Immature granulocytes (myelocytes and metamyelocytes) are found frequently in peripheral blood smears during pregnancy.[46,47] There are no specific data regarding the white cell count during labor and the early puerperium; however, transiently high values (even up to 25×10^9/L) are commonly found.

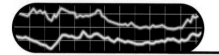
HEMOGLOBIN AND RED BLOOD CELL INDICES

Parameter	Non-pregnant (SD)	12 weeks (SD)	36 weeks (SD)	Postpartum (SD)
Red blood cell count (x 10^{12}/L)	4.688 (0.309)	4.008 (0.247)	3.880 (0.304)	4.493 (0.338)
Hemoglobin concentration (g/dl)	13.30 (0.77)	12.03 (0.70)	11.07 (0.84)	12.69 (0.92)
Hematocrit (L/L)	0.3936 (0.0233)	0.3515 (0.0226)	0.3311 (0.0232)	0.3787 (0.0289)
Mean cell volume (fL)	83.7 (3.1)	86.2 (3.6)	85.0 (5.3)	84.1 (3.8)
Mean cell hemoglobin (pg)	28.39 (1.06)	30.07 (1.16)	28.65 (2.00)	28.23 (1.45)
Mean cell hemoglobin concentration (g/dl)	33.75 (0.68)	34.23 (1.13)	33.46 (0.82)	33.47 (0.93)

(a)

Figure 28 (a) Hemoglobin and red cell indices (mean and SD) from a longitudinal study of women recruited at 12 weeks who delivered after 37 weeks ($n = 24$). No iron or folate supplements were given. 'Non-pregnant' samples were taken 4–6 months post-delivery. Samples were analyzed in a Coulter counter. *Data source:* ref. 45, with permission.

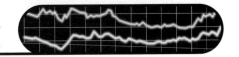

Parameter	Non-pregnant (SD)	12 weeks (SD)	36 weeks (SD)	Postpartum (SD)
Red blood cell count (x 10^{12}/L)	4.621 (0.238)	4.109 (0.227)	4.119 (0.246)	4.370 (0.169)
Hemoglobin concentration (g/dl)	13.42 (0.66)	12.06 (0.57)	12.66 (0.81)	13.03 (0.45)
Hematocrit (L/L)	0.3971 (0.0190)	0.3539 (0.020)	0.3666 (0.020)	0.3880 (0.0123)
Mean cell volume (fL)	85.7 (2.2)	86.0 (3.3)	88.8 (2.9)	88.4 (3.3)
Mean cell hemoglobin (pg)	29.00 (0.77)	29.43 (1.03)	30.76 (1.24)	29.86 (1.20)
Mean cell hemoglobin concentration (g/dl)	33.63 (0.69)	34.05 (1.08)	34.50 (0.82)	33.59 (0.66)

(b)

Figure 28 (b) Hemoglobin and red cell indices (mean and SD) from a longitudinal study of women recruited at 12 weeks who delivered after 37 weeks ($n = 21$). All were given iron and folate supplements from 12 weeks' gestation. 'Non-pregnant' samples were taken 4–6 months post-delivery. Samples were analyzed in a Coulter counter. *Data source:* ref. 45, with permission.

Comment: Hemoglobin concentration falls in the first trimester, whether or not iron and folate supplements are given. Pregnancy-induced hematological changes are still present 6–8 weeks postpartum.

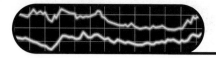

PLATELET COUNT AND INDICES

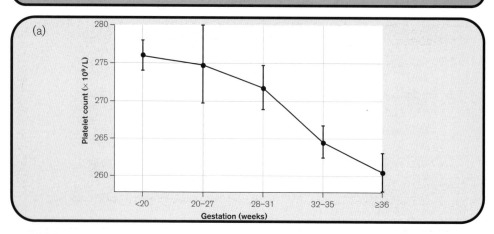

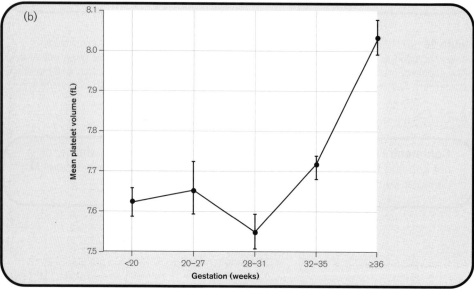

Figure 29 (a) Platelet count and (b) mean platelet volume (mean ± SEM) during pregnancy. The study was largely cross-sectional in design (2881 samples from 2114 women). Samples were analyzed in a Coulter counter. At the end of the study, any patients who had developed hypertension were excluded. *Data source:* ref. 48, with permission, the American College of Obstetrics and Gynecology.

Comment: It has been suggested that there is hyperdestruction of platelets in pregnancy, with a consequent decrease in platelet lifespan. Young platelets are known to be larger than old platelets. Another study[49] of longitudinal design, but with much smaller numbers (*n* = 44) did not find evidence of significant change in the platelet count with gestational age.

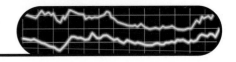

IRON METABOLISM

(a)

Patients	Hb (g/dl)	Serum iron		Transferrin/ TIBC saturation (%)	Serum ferritin (µg/L)
		(µmol/L)	(µg/dl)		
Non-treated (*n* = 30)					
First trimester	12.9	23	129	36	96
Term	12.0	14	78	13	13
Given FeSO₄ (*n* = 82)					
First trimester	12.5	22	123	33	67
Term	12.5	25	140	27	41

(b)

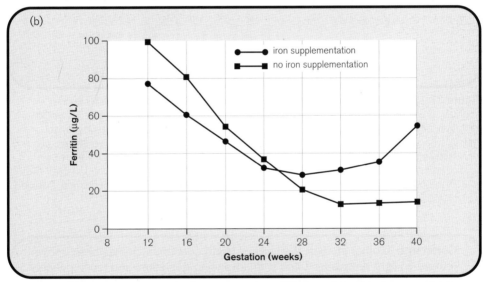

Figure 30 (a) Mean hemoglobin (Hb) and iron indices (TIBC, total iron-binding capacity) from a longitudinal study of women recruited in the first trimester. At the start, 72 were randomized to the 'no treatment' group, but any whose mean hemoglobin level fell below 11 g/dL were prescribed ferrous sulfate 60 mg t.d.s.; thus only 30 progressed through pregnancy without iron supplements. In all subjects studied, serum ferritin levels (b) rose rapidly postpartum, reaching similar values to those found in early pregnancy by 5–8 weeks after delivery (NB: no iron supplements were given following delivery). *Data source:* ref. 50, with permission.

Comment: Iron stores (as indicated by serum ferritin) become depleted during pregnancy, whether or not iron supplements are given.

SERUM AND RED CELL FOLATE

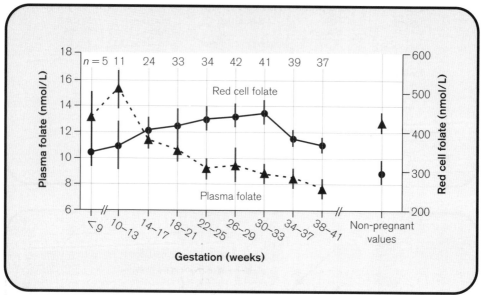

Figure 31 Longitudinal study of plasma and red cell folate levels (mean ± SEM) during singleton pregnancy; all women were taking iron supplements from approximately 12 weeks' gestation, but none took folate supplements ($n = 43$). Samples were taken after overnight fasting, with patients seated. Non-pregnant reference samples were from 50 healthy women (non-lactating) aged 19–37 years, taken 3–5 h following their last meal. None of the women developed anemia during pregnancy (hemoglobin and mean cell volume remained stable). *Data source:* ref. 51, with permission, Munksgaard International Publishers Ltd. Copenhagen, Denmark. *Conversion factor* for folate: mmol/L × 0.044 = µg/dl.

Comment: In other studies, the red cell folate concentration has been shown to have a slight downward trend with advancing gestation, and those patients with a low red cell folate level at the beginning of pregnancy develop megaloblastic anemia in the third trimester.[52] These differences may relate to dietary folate intake. In a cross-sectional study of 155 women, the red cell folate concentration increased with gestation and was significantly higher in those subjects who took supplemental folic acid (1 mg daily) than those who did not (1056 versus 595 nmol/L).[53] Plasma and red cell folate values are similar in pregnant women at term, regardless of their parity.[51] In the 6 weeks following delivery, plasma and red cell folate levels return toward non-pregnant values, although lactation (which constitutes an added folate stress) may delay recovery.[54]

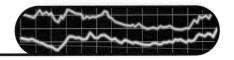

HOMOCYSTEINE

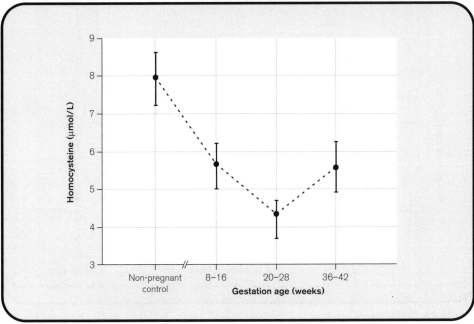

Figure 32 Plasma homocysteine (mean and 95% confidence interval (CI)) levels in a cross-sectional study of 155 normal women in the first, second, and third trimesters of pregnancy and in non-pregnant controls. Homocysteine concentrations were determined by high-pressure liquid chromatography. *Data source:* ref. 53, with permission.

Comment: Plasma homocysteine levels are significantly lower in all trimesters of pregnancy compared to non-pregnant control values. The lowest levels are found in the second trimester. Homocysteine is 70–80% albumin-bound, so these gestational changes mirror those of serum albumin (see Fig. 15). Homocysteine is negatively correlated with red cell folate, and lower concentrations are found in women taking folic acid supplements.[53] Hyperhomocysteinemia, which can result from genetic and environmental factors, is associated with deep venous thrombosis, recurrent miscarriage, abruption, stillbirth, and neural tube defects.

VITAMIN B$_{12}$

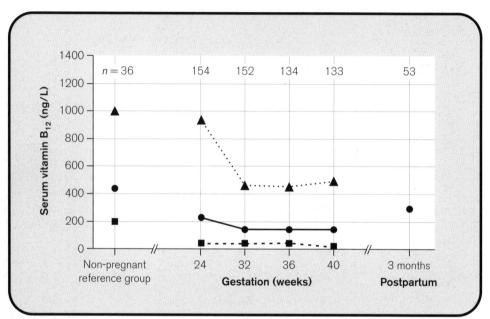

Figure 33 Serum vitamin B$_{12}$ levels (mean and range) measured longitudinally in pregnancy; only 53 of the original group had levels measured postpartum. Non-pregnant reference values were from 36 different women in their child-bearing years. *Data source:* ref. 55, with permission.

Comment: Serum vitamin B$_{12}$ levels fall in the first trimester.[55] They tend to be lower in smokers. Muscle and red cell vitamin B$_{12}$ concentrations also fall during pregnancy; however, vitamin B$_{12}$ absorption does not change.[54]

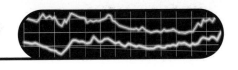

COAGULATION FACTORS

No. of patients		41	48	47	66	62	48	61	61
Weeks		11–15	16–20	21–25	26–30	31–35	36–40	Post-delivery	Postnatal
Factor VII	Mean	111	129	150	158	162	171	134	94
	Range	60–206	68–244	80–280	75–332	84–312	87–336	70–255	52–171
Fibrinogen (g/L)	Mean	3.63	3.65	3.65	3.78	4.17	4.23	4.61	2.65
	Range	2.64–5.00	2.55–5.22	2.53–5.26	2.67–5.35	2.90–6.00	2.90–6.15	2.98–7.14	1.71–4.11
Factor X	Mean	103	111	115	126	123	127	117	90
	Range	62–169	74–166	74–177	78–203	78–194	72–208	72–191	54–149
Factor V	Mean	93	84	82	82	82	85	91	81
	Range	46–188	46–155	36–185	34–214	34–195	39–184	36–233	42–155
Factor II	Mean	125	128	125	124	115	115	112	106
	Range	70–224	75–218	73–214	79–193	74–179	68–194	74–170	68–165
Factor VIII: C	Mean	122	150	141	188	185	212	206	95
	Range	53–283	53–419	44–453	67–528	69–499	79–570	74–569	46–193
Factor VIIIR: Ag	Mean	133	156	167	203	262	376	421	89
	Range	56–318	55–439	66–427	84–492	95–718	133–1064	169–1042	29–272
Factor VIIIR: Ag/VIII: C ratio	Mean	1.09	1.04	1.18	1.08	1.42	1.77	2.05	0.95
	Range	0.43–2.74	0.40–2.72	0.43–3.27	0.41–2.81	0.48–4.21	0.62–5.09	0.71–5.92	0.36–2.52

(Where no units are stated, values are expressed as percentage of standard.)

Figure 34 Coagulation factors (mean and 95% ranges) from a longitudinal study of 72 women (healthy primigravida, or multigravida whose previous pregnancies had been uncomplicated), aged 19–42 years. Post-delivery samples were taken between 6 h and 4 days following delivery (mean 52 h); postnatal samples were taken after 6 weeks. The postnatal samples yielded similar values to those from an age-matched non-pregnant group of women (n = 66). *Data source:* ref. 56, with permission.

Comment: Normal pregnancy is a hypercoagulable state associated with increased levels of factors VII, VIII, and X, and also a very marked increase in fibrinogen levels due to increased synthesis. Factor IX levels rise and factor XI levels fall.[54] Not shown is the increase in fibrinopeptide A, which occurs in the first trimester.

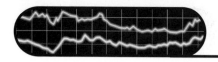

NATURALLY OCCURRING ANTICOAGULANTS AND FIBRINOLYTIC FACTOR

No. of patients		41	48	47	66	62	48	61	61
Weeks		11–15	16–20	21–25	26–30	31–35	36–40	Post-delivery	Postnatal
FDPs (µg/mL)	Mean	1.07	1.06	1.09	1.13	1.28	1.32	1.66	1.04
Fibrinolytic activity (Lysis time in hours)	Min	7.6	7.4	7.3	5.5	4.5	5.6	14.8	17.4
	Max	13.25	13.5	13.75	18.25	22.25	17.8	6.75	5.75
Antithrombin III: C	Mean	85	90	87	94	87	86	87	92
	Range	49–120	46–133	42–132	47–141	42–132	40–132	48–127	38–147
Antithrombin III: Ag	Mean	93	94	93	97	96	93	95	100
	Range	60–126	56–131	56–130	56–138	59–132	50–136	58–133	64–134
α1-Antitrypsin	Mean	124	136	125	146	149	154	172	77
	Range	66–234	86–214	53–295	85–249	89–250	91–260	84–352	44–135
α2-Macroglobulin	Mean	176	178	170	160	157	153	146	142
	Range	100–309	98–323	92–312	88–294	85–292	85–277	81–265	82–245

(Where no units are stated, values are expressed as percentage of standard.)

Figure 35 Naturally occurring concentrations of anticoagulants and fibrinolytic factors (mean and 95% ranges), fibrinolytic activity (full range), and fibrin degradation products (mean values) from a longitudinal study. Patients were those described in Figure 34. *Data source:* ref. 56, with permission.

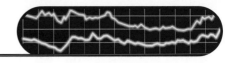

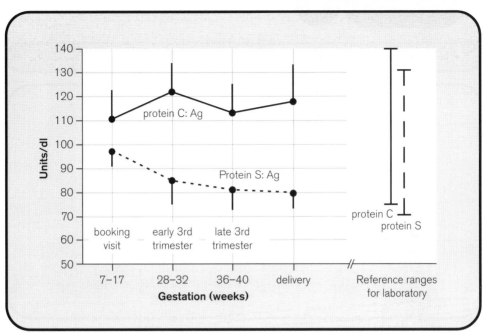

Figure 36 Protein S and C levels (mean and SD) from a longitudinal study in 14 healthy women aged 24–38 years. *Data source:* ref. 57, with permission.

Comment: Free protein S levels fall progressively during pregnancy but remain within the normal reference ranges; protein C levels change little. Antithrombin III levels are stable during pregnancy, fall in labor, and then rise 1 week postpartum.[54] Fibrinolysis is depressed during pregnancy; both fibrinogen and plasminogen levels are elevated, but there are decreased levels of circulating plasminogen activator.[58]

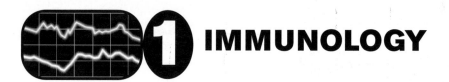

IMMUNOLOGY

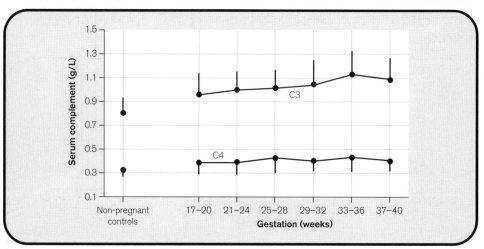

Figure 37 Levels of complement factors C3 and C4 (mean and SD) from a longitudinal study of 147 healthy women, who remained normotensive throughout pregnancy. The control population was 32 normal non-pregnant women, aged 15–41 years, 11 of whom were taking oral contraceptives. *Data source:* ref. 59, with permission.

Comment: Levels of C3 and C4 are significantly elevated during the second and third trimesters of pregnancy. Another cross-sectional study[60] showed elevated levels of C4, but not C3, during the first trimester. Circulating immune complexes are low during pregnancy.[60] There is some disagreement as to whether C3 degradation products are elevated[60] or normal;[61] no longitudinal studies have been done.

MARKERS OF INFLAMMATION

Erythrocyte sedimentation rate (ESR) and C-reactive protein (CRP)

Comment: Values of ESR are high in pregnancy (typically > 30 mm in the first hour) due to elevated levels of plasma globulins and fibrinogen.[62] Thus, ESR cannot be used as a marker for inflammation. Levels of C-reactive protein are undetectable in healthy pregnant women; elevations are due to intercurrent disease.

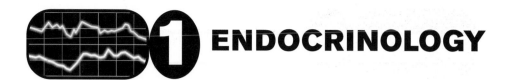

ENDOCRINOLOGY

Total thyroxine (T₄), tri-iodothyronine (T₃), T₃ uptake, and thyroid-binding globulin (TBG)

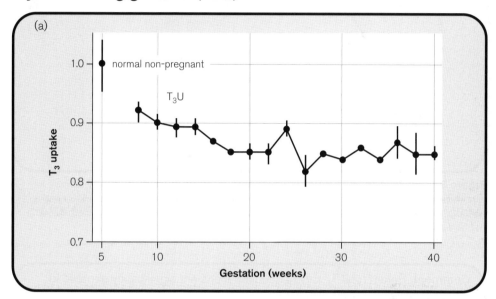

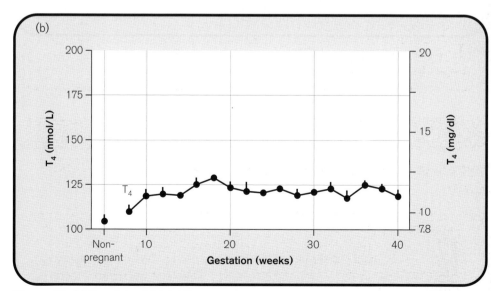

Figure 38 (a) T_3 uptake, (b) total T_4.

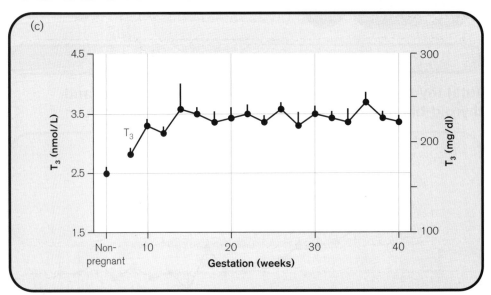

Figure 38 (c) total T_3 (mean ± SEM) from a mostly cross-sectional study of 339 women at various stages of pregnancy; 10–45 were sampled in each 2 week period from 6–40 weeks' gestation. The controls were 40 non-pregnant women of similar age. *Data source:* ref. 63, with permission.

Comment: Serum total T_4 and T_3 concentrations are significantly elevated in pregnancy. The T_3 uptake test is low in pregnancy, indicating unsaturation of TBG. TBG concentrations are doubled by the end of the first trimester, remain elevated throughout pregnancy, and fall slowly in the 6 weeks following delivery.[64]

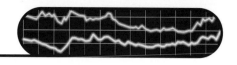

Free T_4, free T_3, and thyroid-stimulating hormone (TSH)

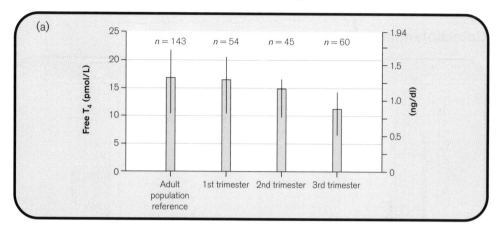

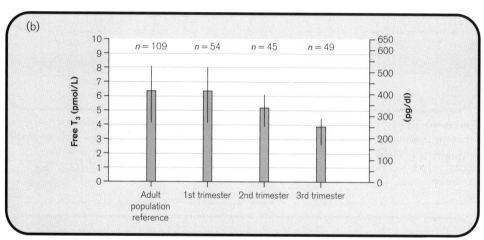

Figure 39 (a) Free T_4 and (b) free T_3 concentrations (mean ± 2 SD) from a cross-sectional study of 159 women attending antenatal clinics; all were free from metabolic illness. The control samples were from 109 patients (male and female), taken from the routine workload of the laboratory (excluding those with thyroid disease, diabetes, cardiac disease, or carcinoma, or patients in a postoperative state). *Data source:* ref. 65, with permission.

Comment: Free T_4 and T_3 concentrations in pregnancy, measured directly (rather than derived from resin uptake measurements) lie within normal non-pregnant ranges, generally.[66] However, a number of different assay methods are available; some yield lower values in late pregnancy.[65] TSH levels, measured by radioimmunoassay, are unchanged in normal pregnancy, although some studies have found low levels toward the end of the first trimester in association with the highest circulating concentrations of human chorionic gonadotropin (hCG).[63]

ADRENAL FUNCTION

Catecholamines

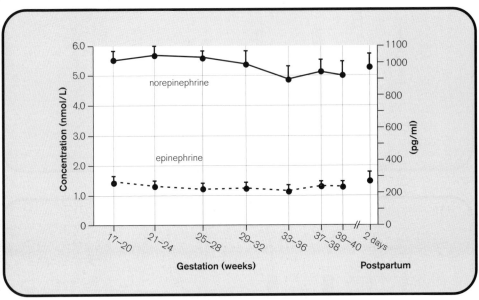

Figure 40 Epinephrine and norepinephrine concentrations (mean and SEM) from a longitudinal study of 52 women, mean age 28 years, who remained normotensive throughout pregnancy; 39 were primigravida. Samples were taken after 20 min of rest in the left lateral position by venepuncture; a radioenzymic method was used for the assays. *Data source:* ref. 67, with permission.

Comment: This study showed a decline in plasma levels of both epinephrine and norepinephrine as pregnancy progressed. Other studies (in which blood samples were taken from indwelling intravenous cannulas) have shown steady levels through pregnancy, with no difference between values during pregnancy and those in the early puerperium.[68] In healthy pregnant women, plasma epinephrine and norepinephrine concentrations show a diurnal pattern, with lowest levels during the night.[69] Urinary vanillomandelic acid (VMA) excretion has not been studied in healthy pregnancies, but is likely to be within the normal adult range.

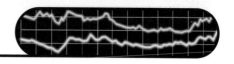

Glucocorticoids

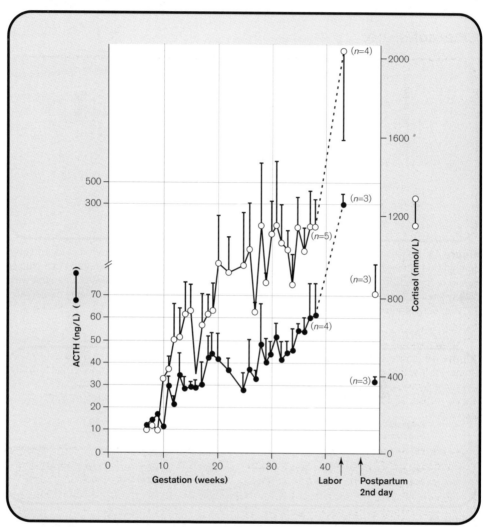

Figure 41 (a) Adrenocorticotropic hormone (ACTH) and cortisol concentrations (mean and SEM) from a longitudinal study of five healthy pregnant women, aged 17–28 years. Blood samples were taken weekly at 0800 to 0900 h after an overnight fast, from early pregnancy until delivery. Samples for ACTH measurement were collected improperly from one woman, and had to be discarded. Samples were also taken from three of these subjects during labor and on the second postpartum day. *Data source:* ref. 70, with permission.

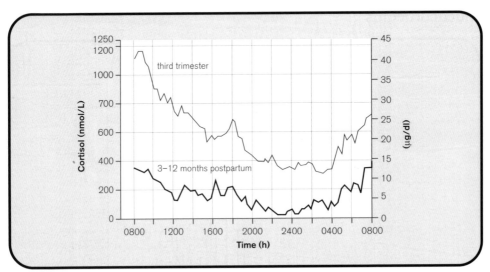

Figure 41 (b) Mean plasma cortisol levels throughout a 24 h study period from a study of seven primigravida in the third trimester and three non-pregnant women, two of whom had been studied during pregnancy. The non-pregnant women were at least 3 months after delivery, and none was breast-feeding or using oral contraceptives. Samples were taken every 20 min. *Data source:* ref. 71, with permission.

	Plasma cortisol (nmol/L)			Free cortisol index	
	Minimum	Mean (in 24-h period)	Maximum	Minimum (in 24-h period)	Maximum
Pregnant third trimester (*n* = 7)	197 (25)	581 (28)	1206 (94)	2.2 (0.3)	15.7 (1.7)
Non-pregnant (*n* = 3)	22 (6)	175 (25)	450 (3)	0.22 (0.05)	5.7 (0.9)

Figure 41 (c) Plasma cortisol levels and free cortisol index (mean and SD) from a study of seven primigravidae in the third trimester and three non-pregnant women, two of whom had been studied during pregnancy. Subjects were those described in Figure 41b. *Data source:* ref. 71, with permission.

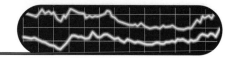

Comment (Figs 41a–41c): The total plasma cortisol level, free plasma cortisol level, and the free cortisol index are increased in pregnancy as compared to the non-pregnant state. ACTH levels during pregnancy are variously reported as remaining within the normal range for non-pregnant subjects, increasing, or decreasing,[70,72] but there is agreement that levels rise with advancing gestation. The rise in ACTH during pregnancy is attributed to placental production of the peptide.[72] Normal diurnal patterns of cortisol (despite overall elevated levels) are found during pregnancy (i.e. lowest values at 2400 h, highest values at 0800 h[71]). The biological half-life of cortisol is increased in pregnancy.[71] Cortisol-binding globulin (CBG) concentrations rise steadily during pregnancy, reaching twice normal values by mid-gestation.[73] Cortisol production rate during pregnancy has been described as being depressed[74] or elevated.[71] The urinary free cortisol level more than doubles during pregnancy.[75] Plasma cortisol levels measured at 0800 h following 1 mg of dexamethasone given orally at 2300 h the previous evening suppress to below 139 nmol/L or 5 μg/dL (a normal response);[76] however, urinary cortisol levels do not suppress as much in pregnant as in non-pregnant subjects.[72] The cortisol response to an ACTH challenge (Synacthen test) is unchanged in pregnancy.[77]

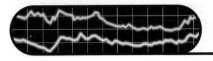

PROLACTIN

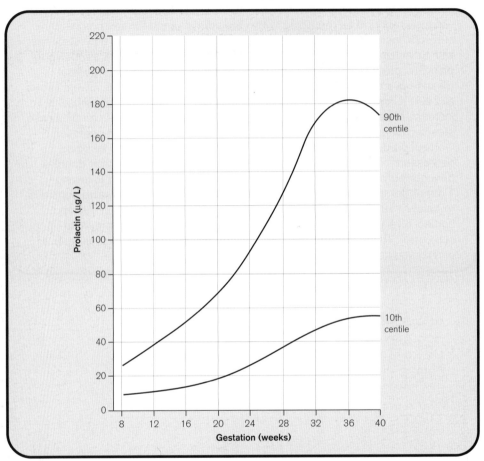

Figure 42 Serum prolactin levels (10th and 90th centiles) from a mostly cross-sectional study of 839 women with uncomplicated singleton pregnancies between 8 and 40 weeks' gestation; a total of 980 blood samples were taken. All samples were collected between 0900 and 1100 h. Any women who developed a pregnancy complication was rejected from the normal series. *Data source:* ref. 78, with permission.

Comment: Prolactin concentrations increase 10–20-fold during the course of pregnancy. There is a normal circadian rhythm, with a nocturnal rise.[79] In labor, there is an acute fall in levels, then a postpartum surge during the first 2 h following delivery;[80] these changes are not seen in women undergoing elective cesarean deliveries. Prolactin levels approach the normal range 2–3 weeks after delivery in non-lactating women, but remain elevated in those who breast-feed their infants.[81]

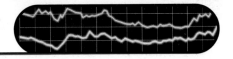

CALCIUM METABOLISM

Total and ionized calcium, magnesium, albumin, parathyroid hormone (PTH), calcitonin, and vitamin D

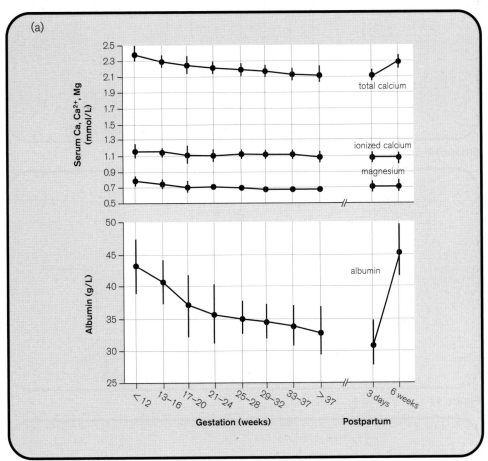

Figure 43 (a) Total and ionized calcium, magnesium, and albumin levels (mean ± SD) from a longitudinal study of 30 women, recruited in the first trimester and studied at intervals of 4 weeks. Samples were also taken on the third postpartum day and during the sixth postpartum week. The subjects ranged in age from 19 to 33 years; 20 were primigravidae. Samples were collected by venepuncture after an overnight fast. *Data source:* ref. 82, with permission. Conversion factors: calcium, nmol/L × 4 = mg/dL; magnesium, mmol/L × 2.4 = mg/dL.

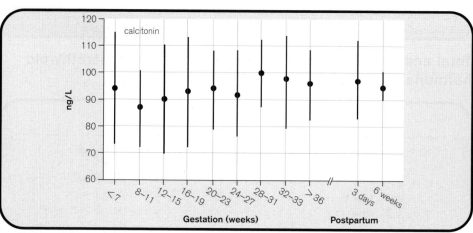

Figure 43 (b) Calcitonin.

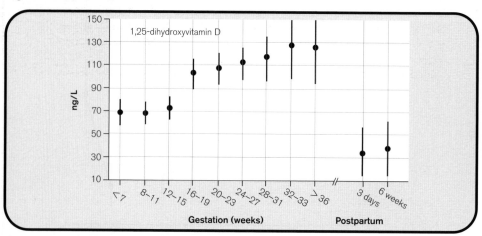

Figure 43 (c) 1,25-dihydroxy-vitamin D.

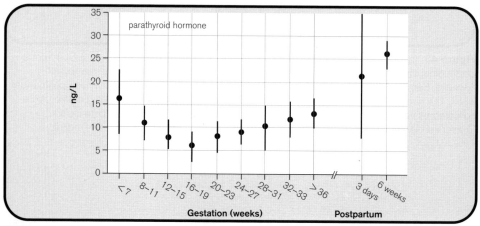

Figure 43 (d) Parathyroid hormone (PTH).

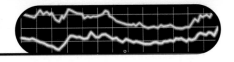

Figure 43 (b) Calcitonin, (c) 1,25-dihydroxy-vitamin D and (d) PTH concentrations (mean ± SD) from a longitudinal study of 20 women, aged 22–34 years, 12 of whom were nulliparous. All had uncomplicated pregnancies of more than 38 weeks' gestation. The only medication they received was ferrous sulfate. Blood samples were taken in the morning after an overnight fast. Samples were collected at intervals of 4 weeks, the first being taken before 7 weeks' gestation, and also on the third postpartum day and during the sixth postpartum week. *Data source:* ref. 83, with permission.

Comment (Figs 43a to 43d): total serum calcium levels decline during pregnancy, in association with the fall in serum albumin levels; however, ionized calcium levels remain constant. Serum intact PTH levels are lower in pregnancy than at 6 weeks postpartum; they reach their nadir in mid-pregnancy. A menstrual cyclicity in PTH has also been noted, with higher values corresponding to times of increased estrogen secretion.[82] Calcitonin levels are not significantly altered in pregnancy. 1,25-Dihydroxy-vitamin D levels rise with advancing gestation, and are significantly higher than during the puerperium. Some 1α-hydroxylation of 25-hydroxy-vitamin D has been demonstrated in the placenta to account for this rise and the consequent suppression of PTH.[83]

PLACENTAL BIOCHEMISTRY

Plasma protein A (PAPP-A)

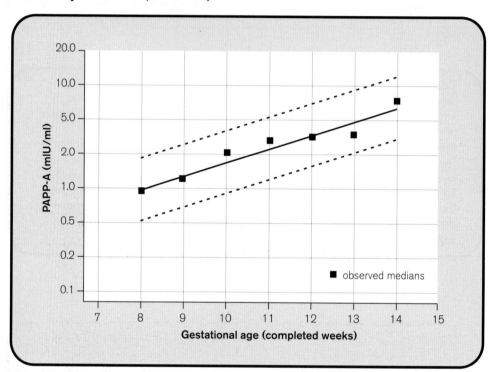

Figure 44 PAPP-A levels in maternal serum (median, 0.5 × median and 2 × median) from a cross-sectional study of 379 healthy women between 8 and 14 weeks' gestation. As these women had been selected to match 77 women whose fetuses had been found to have Down's syndrome, they were of median age 39 years (10th and 90th centiles, 34 and 42 years, respectively). *Data source:* ref. 84, with permission.

Comment: PAPP-A and free β-hCG are useful markers for discriminating Down's syndrome from normal pregnancies at 8–14 weeks' gestation. PAPP-A levels are lower in affected pregnancies than normal (particularly so at 11 weeks' gestation or less).[84,85]

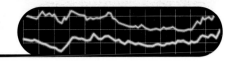

Serum α-fetoprotein (SAFP)

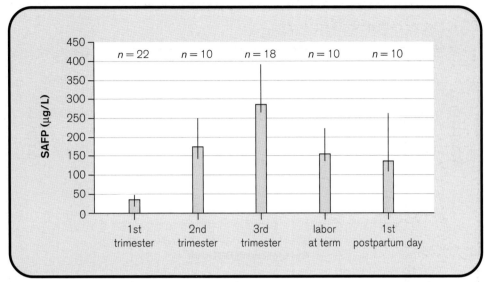

Figure 45 SAFP levels (median and IQ range) from a cross-sectional study; samples from women in labor and on the first postpartum day were paired. SAFP was measured by radioimmunoassay. *Data source:* ref. 86, with permission.

Comment: In the second trimester, SAFP rises by approximately 15% per week.[87] Reference ranges for SAFP in the second trimester are established by individual screening laboratories for their own population, and are usually expressed as multiples of the median (MoM) for gestation. Twin pregnancies are associated with SAFP levels approximately twice as high as those of singleton pregnancies.[87] Maternal weight is inversely related to SAFP levels, probably due to the dilutional effect of a larger vascular compartment.[87]

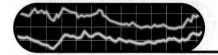

Human chorionic gonadotropin (hCG)

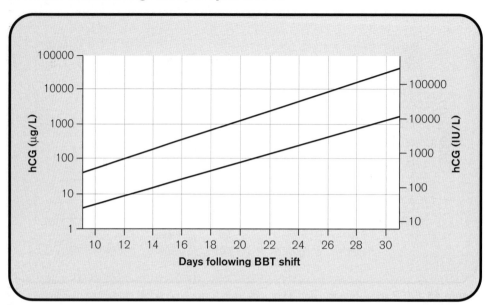

Figure 46 (a) Serum values of the β-subunit of hCG (95% CI) measured in 189 women who subsequently had successful pregnancies (total of 280 samples analyzed). They were patients in an infertility clinic and were keeping basal body temperature (BBT) charts to indicate the timing of ovulation. Some conceptions were spontaneous; other patients were treated with clomiphene citrate, human menopausal gonadotropin, and/or hCG (a single injection of 5000 IU to induce ovulation). A radioimmunoassay was used for β-hCG. *Data source:* ref. 88, with permission.

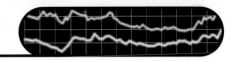

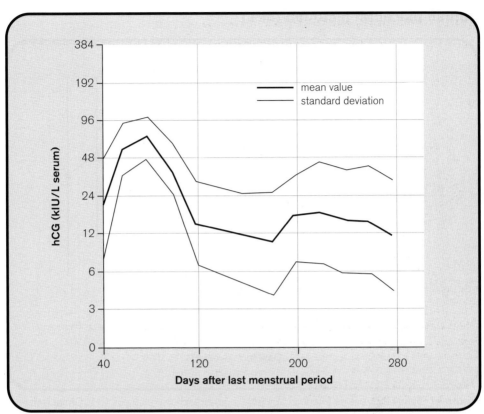

Figure 46 (b) Total serum hCG (mean ± SD) from a longitudinal study of 20 healthy women. The first samples were drawn as early in pregnancy as possible, with subsequent samples every 3–4 weeks; the last sample was taken during labor. Samples were classified into groups with a class interval of 30 days. hCG was determined by radioimmunoassay; the international hCG standard was used as a reference. *Data source:* ref. 89, with permission.

Comment: The mean doubling time of β-hCG is 2.2 days ± 1.0 (2 SD).[88] Low hCG values which do not double within this range are associated with ectopic pregnancies or spontaneous abortions.[88] Women with male fetuses have significantly lower hCG levels than do those with female fetuses.[89]

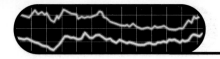

Human placental lactogen (hPL)

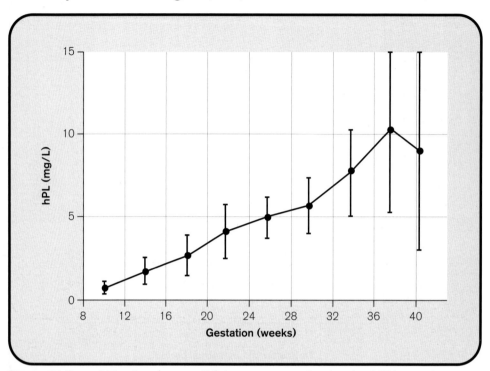

Figure 47 Serum hPL values (mean ± SD) from a cross-sectional study of 151 normal women with singleton pregnancies attending the antenatal clinic. hPL was measured by radioimmunoassay. *Data source:* ref. 90, with permission, the American College of Obstetricians and Gynecologists.

Comment: hPL levels in women with multiple pregnancies are outside these ranges; however, if values are corrected for predicted placental weight then they are appropriate for gestational age.[90] Four hours after delivery of the placenta, plasma hPL is virtually undetectable; the half-life of hPL in the plasma is 21–23 min.[91]

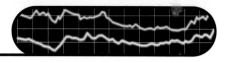

Estriol (E₃)

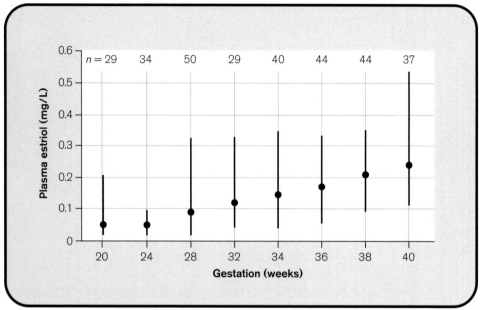

Figure 48 Plasma E$_3$ (mean and range) from a cross-sectional study in women with uncomplicated pregnancies. Plasma E$_3$ was measured by a fluorometric method. *Data source: ref. 92, with permission.*

Comment: The normal range of plasma E$_3$ in pregnancy is wide. In order to assess the significance of values outside this range, trends should be studied over several days.

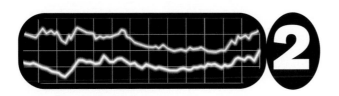

FETAL
VALUES

PHYSIOLOGY
BIOCHEMISTRY
HEMATOLOGY
ENDOCRINOLOGY

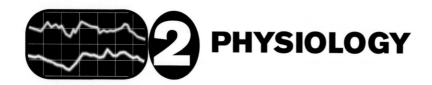

2 PHYSIOLOGY

EARLY EMBRYONIC STRUCTURES

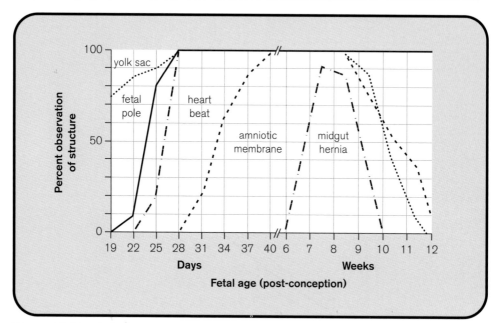

Figure 49 Visualization by ultrasound of yolk sac, fetal pole, heart beat, amniotic membrane, and midgut hernia from a longitudinal study of 39 women with known dates of ovulation; most were patients from an assisted conception unit. They were scanned using a vaginal probe weekly, once pregnancy had been confirmed, starting as early as 18 days post-conception. Five subjects had twin pregnancies. *Data source:* ref. 93, Copyright University of Bristol with permission.

Comment: Transvaginal ultrasound scanning yields better images in the first trimester than does transabdominal scanning. By 28 days post-conception, fetal viability may be confirmed by visualization of a heart beat. The fetal heart rate increases from 90 to 145 beats/min by 7 weeks post-conception.[93]

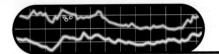

BIOMETRY

Crown–rump length (CRL)

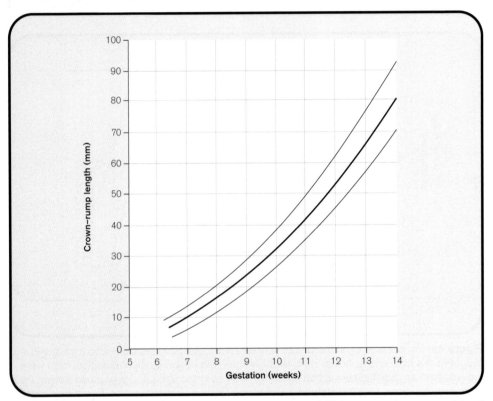

Figure 50 CRL (mean ± 2 SD) from a cross-sectional study of 334 women who were certain of the date of their last menstrual period and had normal regular menstrual cycles. The study covered the time period from 6 to 14 weeks after the last menstrual period. A transabdominal ultrasound technique was used, and the longest length of fetal echoes was found and measured. *Data source:* ref. 94, with permission.

Comment: CRL measurements can only be used effectively in the first trimester. Other studies have found very similar values for CRL; measurements are not influenced by maternal age, height, or parity.[95] In a smaller, longitudinal study CRL was found to be significantly smaller in female than male fetuses.[95] No differences have been found in CRL measurements between Asian and European patients.[96]

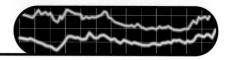
Nuchal translucency (NT)

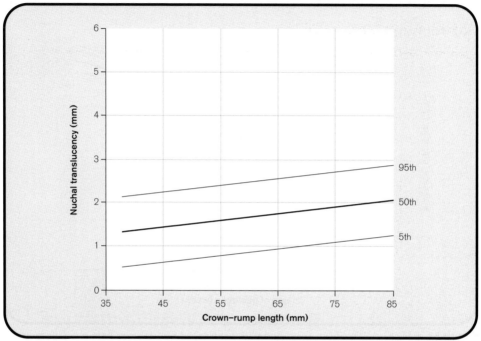

Figure 51 NT measurements (5th, 50th, and 95th centiles) from a cross-sectional study of 20 217 chromosomally normal fetuses examined at 10–14 weeks' gestation. Most examinations were done with transabdominal ultrasound, and all operators were carefully trained in the technique prior to the study. A sagittal section of the fetus was obtained perpendicular to the ultrasound beam, allowing measurement of CRL as well as the maximum thickness of the subcutaneous translucency between skin and soft tissue overlying the cervical spine.[97] Care was taken to avoid confusion between fetal skin and amnion, both of which appear as thin membranes. *Data source:* ref. 98, with permission.

Comment: There is a strong association between abnormal fluid collections in the cervical region (as shown by increased NT measurements) and chromosomal abnormalities. An upper limit of normal may be set at 2.5 or 3.0 mm when using these measurements as a screening test for,[98,99] but it is preferable to use the 95th centile of NT as plotted against CRL, since measurements increase with gestational age.[98]

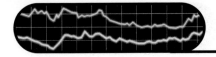

Biparietal diameter (BPD)

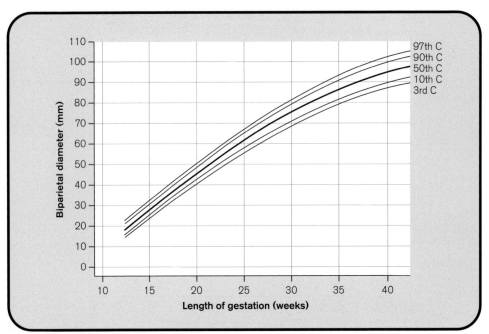

Figure 52 BPD (3rd, 10th, 50th, 90th, and 97th centiles) of 594 fetuses from a prospective cross-sectional study of 663 women with singleton pregnancies carried out in London. Each fetus was measured only once between 12 and 42 weeks' gestation for the purpose of the study. All women had certain menstrual dates, and their menstrual and ultrasound age at 18–22 weeks' gestation did not differ by more than 10 days. The study population consisted of 75% Western European and 25% Afro-Caribbean women. No women had disease or medication likely to affect fetal growth (e.g. diabetes, hypertension, renal disease). Measurements from two fetuses subsequently found to have abnormal karyotypes were excluded from the study. BPD measurements were made in the axial plane of the skull at the level where the continuous midline echo is broken by the cavum septum pellucidum in the anterior third. Measurements presented are those from the proximal edge of the skull closest to the transducer to the proximal edge of the deep border (i.e. outer–inner edges of bone). The statistical methods used to derive graphs and tables from the raw data are described in detail. *Data source:* refs 100 and 101, with permission.

Comment: Other large studies are in close agreement with these measurements.[102,103] Information about growth in BPD is available from a longitudinal study of BPD.[104] Charts and graphs are also available for outer–outer BPD measurements,[101] and regression equations are given for both parameters. There are likely to be some racial differences in fetal measurements, so it is recommended that charts or centile graphs appropriate to the population be used. A small study found no significant differences between Asian and European women living in the same city.[96]

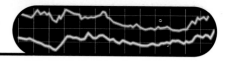

Head circumference (HC)

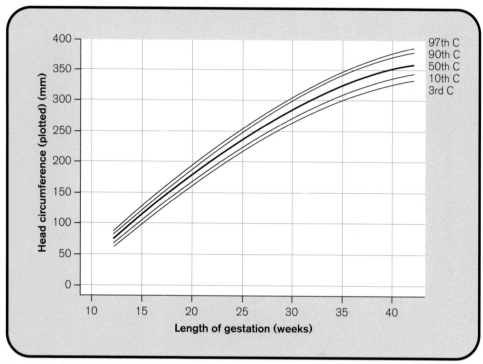

Figure 53 HC (3rd, 10th, 50th, 90th and 97th centiles) from a prospective cross-sectional study of 594 fetuses, as described in Figure 52. HC was measured directly by tracing around the perimeter of the skull in the same plane as used for BPD measurements. *Data source:* refs 100 and 101, with permission.

Comment: HC measurements as derived from the biparietal and occipitofrontal diameters are also available,[101,102] as well as the regression equations for each parameter. Other studies have yielded very similar data, but there are some differences in the late third trimester.[102,105] These have been attributed to patient recruitment characteristics (whether only women delivering at term were included in the study) and the numbers of ultrasound operators used in collection of data. HC measurements are particularly useful in the assessment of gestational age where there is an abnormality of fetal head shape, e.g. dolicocephaly.

Abdominal circumference (AC)

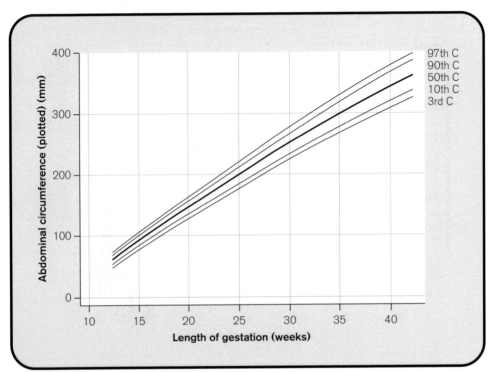

Figure 54 AC (3rd, 10th, 50th, 90th, and 97th centiles) from 610 fetuses, in the prospective cross-sectional study described in Figure 52. The fetal abdomen was measured in a transverse section, with the spine and descending aorta posteriorly, the umbilical vein in the anterior third, and the stomach bubble in the same plane. Care was taken to ensure that the section was as close as possible to circular, perpendicular to the spine. The circumference was measured by tracing around the perimeter. *Data source*: refs 100 and 106, with permission.

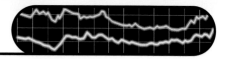

Comment: AC variability increases with gestational age as shown by widening of the centiles. Other large studies are in close agreement[103,107,108] with these values. Studies where all women delivered at term did not find flattening of the growth velocity curves in late pregnancy.[109,110] Some of the discrepancies are due to differences in mathematical curve-fitting techniques applied to the experimental data, as well as to differences in the design of the studies and numbers of subjects and operators involved. AC is not a good measurement for confirmation of gestational age, but rather for assessment of size (e.g. in relation to head and limb measurements). A method has been described[107] for assigning Z-scores to measurements, so that deviation from median values can be expressed without graphical presentation of the data and compared between subjects or between the same subject at different times. Regression equations for AC, both plotted and those derived from abdominal diameter measurements, are described.[106,107]

Femur length (FL)

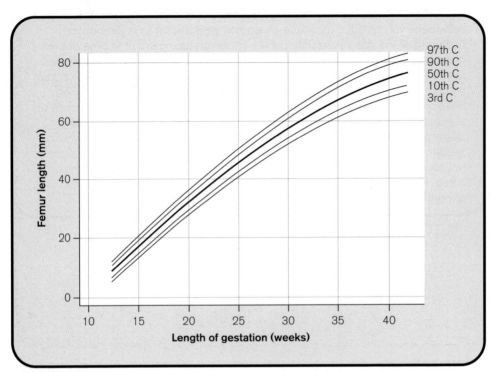

Figure 55 FL (3rd, 10th, 50th, 90th, and 97th centiles) from 649 fetuses, in the prospective cross-sectional study described in Figure 52. The femur was identified and the transducer rotated until the full femoral diaphysis was seen in a plane almost at right angles to the ultrasound beam. The measurement was made from one end of the diaphysis to the other, disregarding any curvature and ignoring the distal femoral epiphysis. *Data source*: refs 100 and 111, with permission.

Comment: Other cross-sectional studies of FL provide very similar measurements,[103,107] although one has wider centiles in late pregnancy.[112] This is likely to be due to a difference in the statistical approach to the calculation of centiles from the regression line. Regression equations are available.[103,107,111]

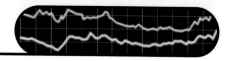

Limb bone lengths

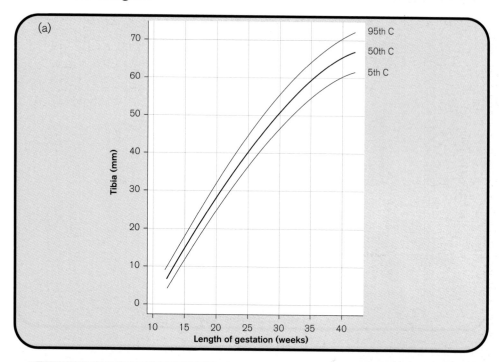

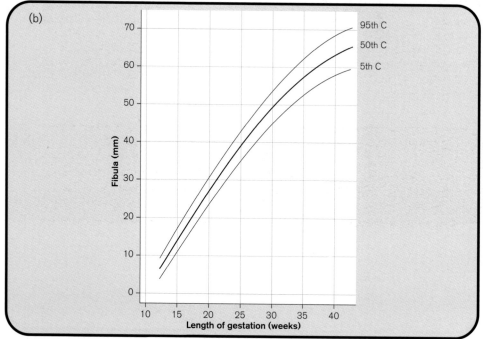

Figure 56 Lengths of (a) tibia, (b) fibula.

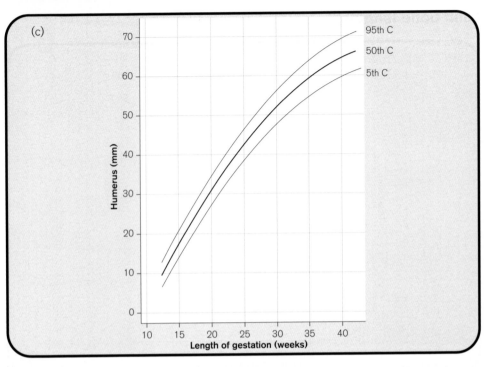

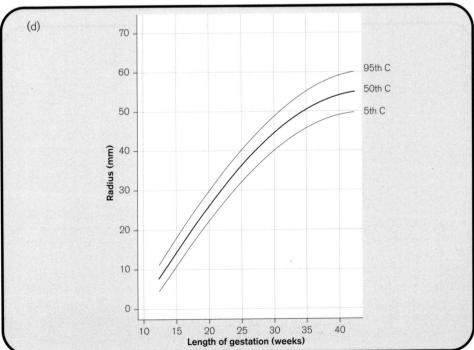

Figure 56 Lengths of (c) humerus, (d) radius.

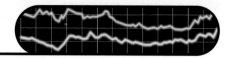

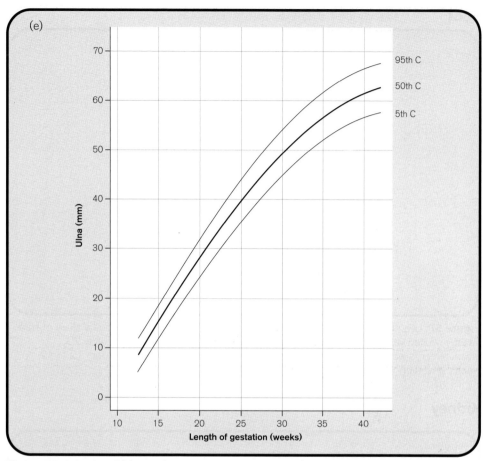

(e)

Figure 56 Lengths of (e) ulna (5th, 50th, and 95th centiles) from a cross-sectional study of 669 healthy women with singleton pregnancies. Any who subsequently delivered an infant with an abnormal karyotype, significant malformation, or any other disease was excluded from the analysis. In all women, menstrual dating was certain, and there was agreement between menstrual age and ultrasound dates at the time of the initial scan. Approximately 20 measurements were obtained for each parameter for each week of gestation from 12 to 42 weeks. *Data source:* ref. 113, with permission.

Comment: All limb bones show linear growth from 13 to 25 weeks; thereafter growth is non-linear. Other studies have confirmed these findings.[114] Good agreement has been found between ultrasound and X-ray measurements of limb bone lengths. Tables are available to allow assessment of gestational age from measurement of limb bone lengths.[115] This use of limb bone measurements should be distinguished from tables or graphs of normal measurements at known gestational age which allow assessment of possible skeletal dysplasias.[113,116]

Foot

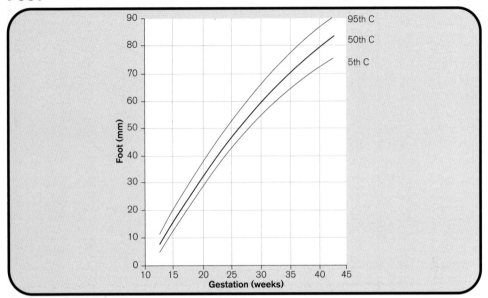

Figure 57 Length of foot (5th, 50th, and 95th centiles) from the cross-sectional study of 669 healthy women with singleton pregnancies, described in Figure 56. Approximately 20 measurements were obtained for each variable for each week of pregnancy from 12 to 42 weeks' gestation. *Data source:* ref. 113, with permission.

Kidney

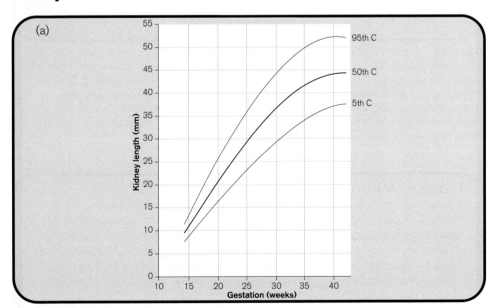

Figure 58 (a)

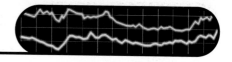

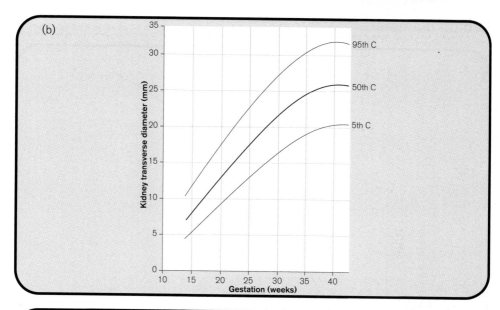

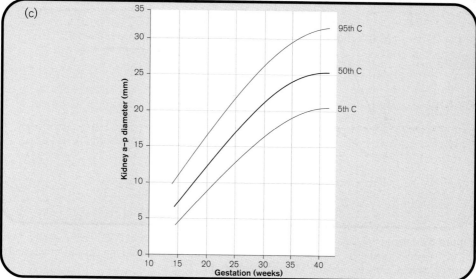

Figure 58 Kidney measurements (5th, 50th, and 95th centiles) from the cross-sectional study of 669 healthy women with singleton pregnancies, described in Figure 56. Approximately 20 measurements were obtained for each variable for each week of pregnancy from 12 to 42 weeks' gestation. *Data source:* ref. 113, with permission.

Comment: The ratio of the transverse renal circumference to the abdominal circumference (in a section at the level of the umbilical vein) is a simple way of assessing normal kidney size; values are 0.27–0.30 from 17 weeks' gestation to term.[117]

Orbital diameters

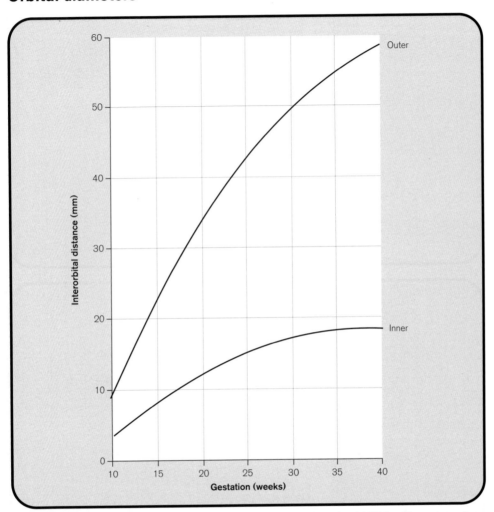

Figure 59 Interorbital distance (mean) from a cross-sectional study of 180 healthy women from 22 to 40 weeks' gestation. A scan plane was obtained which transected the occiput, orbits, and nasal processes. *Data source:* ref. 118, with permission.

Comment: Outer-orbital diameter (IOD) is closely related to BPD. It is a useful measurement when the fetal position precludes accurate measurement of BPD.

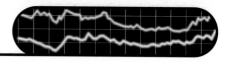

Cerebral ventricles

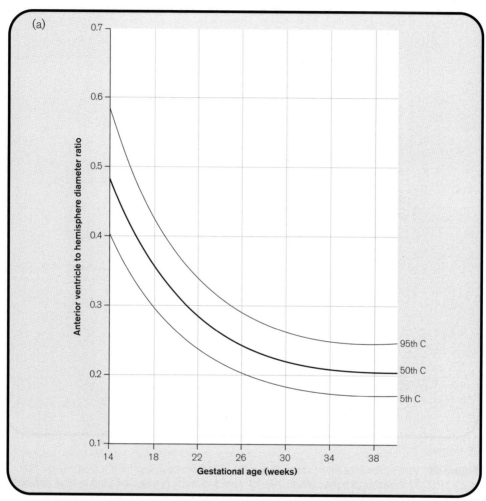

Figure 60 (a) Anterior horn.

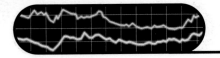
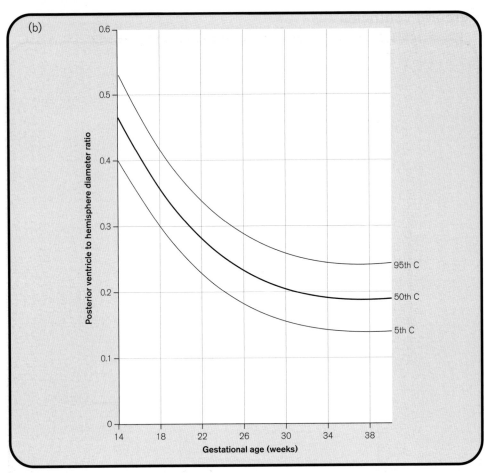

(b) Posterior horn.

Figure 60 Ventriculohemispheric ratios (5th, 50th, and 95th centiles) from a cross-sectional study of 1040 singleton pregnancies at 14–40 weeks' gestation, selected from a large database. All women had known last menstrual period dates with a cycle length of 26–30 days and suffered no pregnancy complications. Only data from structurally normal fetuses who were liveborn at 37 weeks' gestation or later and who had birth weights between the 3rd and 97th centile for gestation were included. For each week, measurements from 40 fetuses were obtained. Each fetus only contributed measurements to the data pool on one occasion. Measurement of the anterior horn (a) of the lateral cerebral ventricle was made in a transverse axial plane of the fetal head (as for BPD or HC measurements), from the lateral wall of the anterior horn to the midline. Posterior horn measurements (b) were made from the medial to the lateral walls of the posterior horn. Hemispheric measurements were made from the mid-line to the inner border of the skull. *Data source:* ref. 103, with permission, Blackwell Science Limited.

Comment: The most reliable measurements of the ventricular system are made using the frontal horns of the lateral cerebral ventricles, as they are the easiest to identify. As a general rule, ventricular diameter should be less than 10 mm.

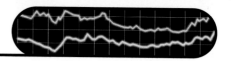

Cerebellum

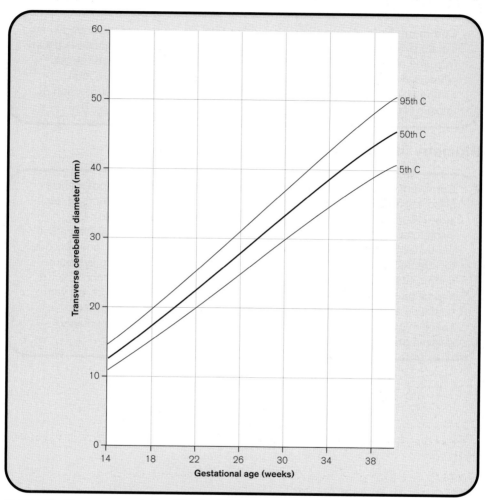

Figure 61 Transverse cerebellar diameter (5th, 50th, and 95th centiles) from the cross-sectional study of 1040 singleton pregnancies described in Figure 60. Measurements were made in the suboccipitobregmatic plane of the fetal head. *Data source:* ref. 103, with permission, Blackwell Science Limited.

Comment: The cerebellum may be visualized as early as 10–11 weeks' gestation. Other studies have found similar measurements.[119]

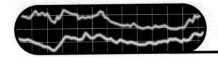
Other fetal measurements

> **Comment:** Normal ranges for many other fetal structures are described in the literature. Each may be useful under certain circumstances. Attention is drawn to charts of *liver length*, useful in the assessment of isoimmunized fetuses where liver length has been shown to be inversely correlated with fetal hemoglobin levels.[120] *Fetal ear* measurements are helpful in the detection of fetuses with abnormal karyotypes.[121,122]

Biometry in multiple gestations

> **Comment:** A longitudinal study of 35 healthy women with twin pregnancies failed to find clinically important differences between measurements of fetal size (HC, BPD, limb bone lengths, etc.) in twins, as compared to singletons.[123,124] Earlier studies[125,126] suggested that BPD measurements in the third trimester were reduced in twins, although HC was not, possibly due to intrauterine crowding. A study of 103 twin gestations, yielding live born, normal infants (which excluded any twin pairs where there was more than 5 mm difference in BPD) found that AC measurements did not increase with gestation at the same rate as singletons.[126] This latter study proposed specific 'twin' growth charts. Studies in normal triplet pregnancies found delay in growth patterns after mid-gestation.[127]

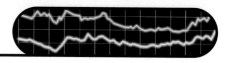

Birth weight

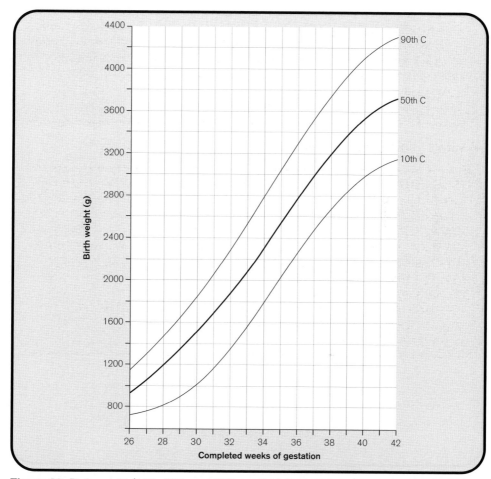

Figure 62 Birth weight (10th, 50th, and 90th centiles) from analysis of 41 718 singleton births in Nottingham, UK, between 1986 and 1991. All women had dates confirmed by ultrasound measurements (CRL up to 13 weeks' gestation, BPD thereafter) before 24 weeks' gestation, and they delivered between 168 and 300 days' gestation. The population was of mixed ethnicity. *Data source:* ref. 128, with permission.

Comment: This study differs from previous ones[129,130] (which did not have ultrasound confirmation of gestational age) in that it found continued increase, rather than flattening, of the birth weight curves toward term. Birth weights of preterm infants (≤32 weeks' gestation) were found to be negatively skewed, consistent with the observation that growth-restricted babies may be born earlier than those of appropriate size.[128] Birth weight is also dependent on ethnic origin, altitude, socioecononomic factors, maternal size, birth order, and maternal cigarette smoking.[128,131,132] All the studies here described are for singletons; different ranges apply to infants from multiple pregnancies.

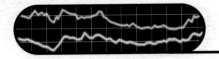
Weight estimated from ultrasound measurements

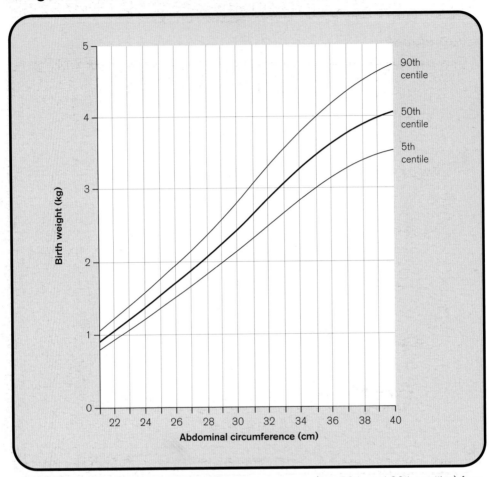

Figure 63 Weight estimated from ultrasound measurements (5th, 50th, and 90th centiles) from a study of 138 women, who had an ultrasound examination within 48 h of delivery for the measurement of fetal AC. The actual birth weights were compared with the AC measurements and a polynomial equation derived to describe the relationship. *Data source:* ref. 133, with permission.

Comment: Equations have also been derived for estimating fetal weight from various combinations of ultrasonic measurements (AC, BPD, HC, and FL)[134,135] which are claimed to be more accurate than those based on AC measurements alone.

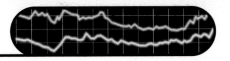

AMNIOTIC FLUID

Total volume

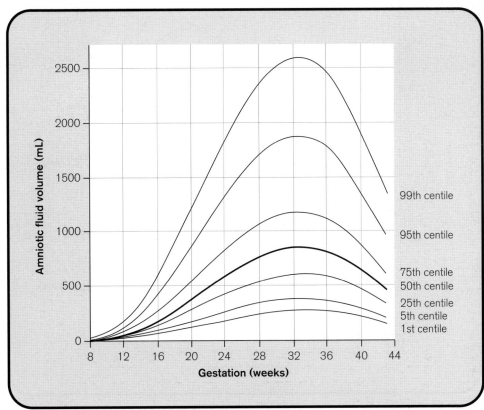

Figure 64 Total amniotic fluid volume (1st, 5th, 25th, 50th, 75th, 95th, and 99th centiles). Composite analysis of 12 published reports of amniotic fluid volume in human pregnancy, totaling 705 measurements. Amniotic fluid volumes were either measured directly at the time of hysterotomy or indirectly using an indicator dilution technique. Only healthy pregnancies were included; any complicated by fetal death or anomaly, or by maternal disease were excluded. *Data source:* ref. 136, with permission.

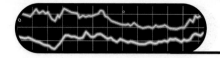
Amniotic fluid index (AFI)

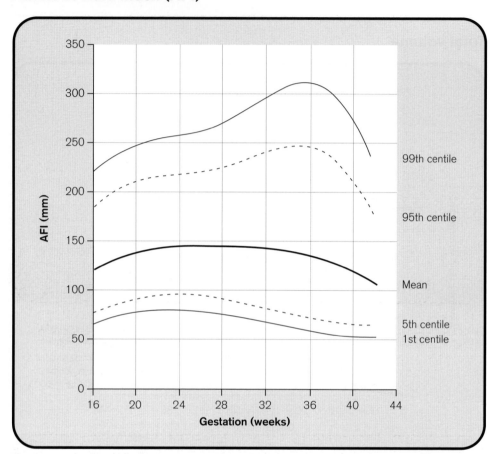

Figure 65 AFI (1st, 5th, 50th, 95th, and 99th centiles) from a prospective study of 791 patients. Any who did not have a normal pregnancy outcome (i.e. infant born at term, between 10th and 90th centile for birth weight, with 5 min Apgar score above 6, and without congenital anomaly) were subsequently excluded. Ultrasound imaging was performed and the uterus divided into four quadrants along the sagittal midline and midway up the fundus. AFI was calculated as the sum of the deepest vertical dimension (in millimeters) of the amniotic fluid pocket in each quadrant of the uterus. *Data source:* ref. 137, with permission.

Comment: AFI rises to a plateau between 22 and 39 weeks' gestation of 700–850 mL. This corresponds to an AFI of 140–150 mm. After term, there is a significant decline in AFI.

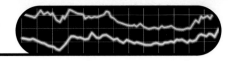

Pressure

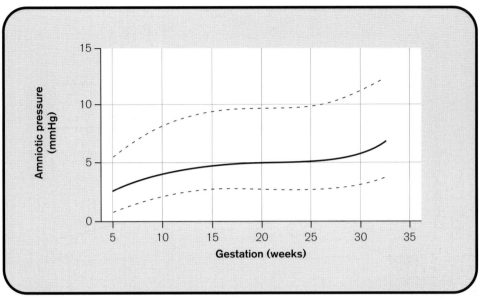

Figure 66 Amniotic fluid pressure (mean and 95% CI) from a cross-sectional study of 171 singleton pregnancies, subsequently shown to have normal karyotype, in whom amniotic fluid volume was subjectively assessed as normal on ultrasonic appearances. All patients were scheduled to undergo a transamniotic invasive procedure for diagnostic reasons or else were to undergo therapeutic termination of pregnancy. Amniotic fluid pressure was measured using a manometry technique referenced to the top of the maternal abdomen. *Data source:* ref. 138, with permission.

Comment: Amniotic fluid pressure rises with gestation, although there is a mid-trimester plateau of 4–5 mmHg. Pressure was not influenced by parity or maternal age and was similar in twin and singleton pregnancies.[138]

Osmolality

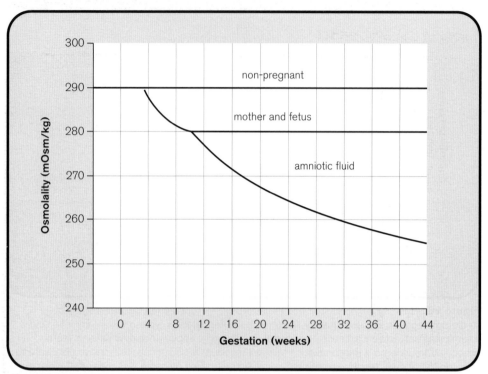

Figure 67 Amniotic fluid osmolality (mean) from a composite analysis of six published reports of amniotic fluid osmolality. *Data source:* ref. 139, with permission, Cambridge University Press.

Comment: In early pregnancy the composition of amniotic fluid is consistent with a transudate of maternal or fetal plasma.[140] The fetal skin becomes keratinized by mid-pregnancy and the amniotic fluid solute concentrations decrease as fetal urine becomes more dilute.[140] Thus there is an osmotic gradient between amniotic fluid and both maternal and fetal plasma.

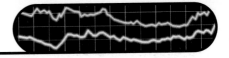

Cardiac circumference

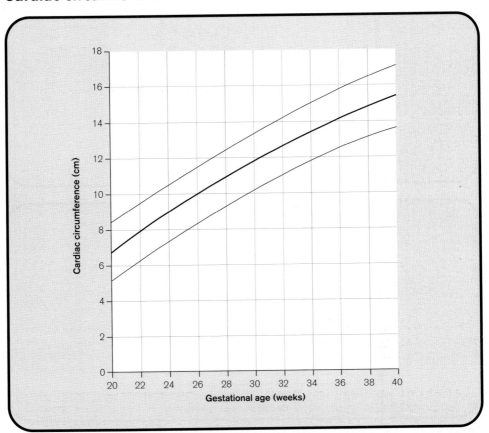

Figure 68 Cardiac circumference (mean and 95% CI) from a longitudinal study of 45 healthy women with known menstrual dates, confirmed by early ultrasound scan. They were recruited prior to 20 weeks' gestation and scanned every 4 weeks. Fetal cardiac and thoracic circumferences were measured in a transverse plane through the chest at the level of the four-chamber view of the fetal heart. *Data source:* ref. 141, with permission.

Comment: The cardiac:thoracic circumference ratio is normally approximately 0.5 (95% CI: at 20 weeks' gestation, 0.40–0.58; at 30 weeks, 0.44–0.60; at 40 weeks, 0.46–0.65).[141]

Ventricular dimensions

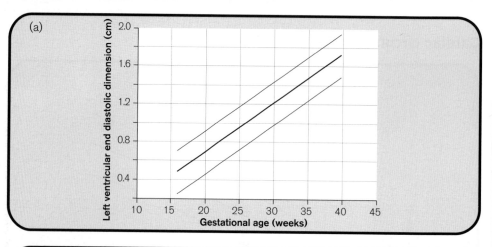

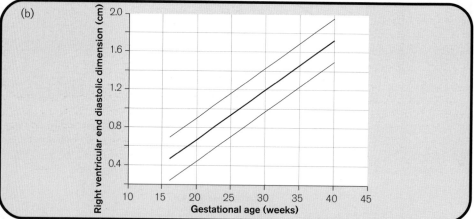

Figure 69 End-diastolic dimensions of (a) the left ventricle and (b) the right ventricle (regression line and 95% prediction interval) from a cross-sectional study of 117 normal women between 16 and 41 weeks' gestation. All fetuses were anatomically normal, and their gestational age had been confirmed by first trimester ultrasound measurements. A four-chamber view of the heart was obtained in a transverse plane through the fetal chest. The transducer was then adjusted so that the intraventricular septum was perpendicular to the ultrasound beam. In this view, transverse endocardial–endocardial dimensions of both ventricles were measured just below the valves, at the end of diastole. *Data source:* ref. 142, with permission, Excerpta Medica Inc.

Comment: This study found narrower confidence intervals for cardiac measurements than earlier ones.[143] This was attributed to improved resolution of newer ultrasound equipment and the use of imaging planes perpendicular to the ultrasound plane (which reduces lateral resolution error). There was close correlation between measurements made between two different observers in this study.

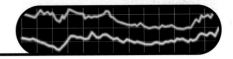

Ventricular and septal wall thickness

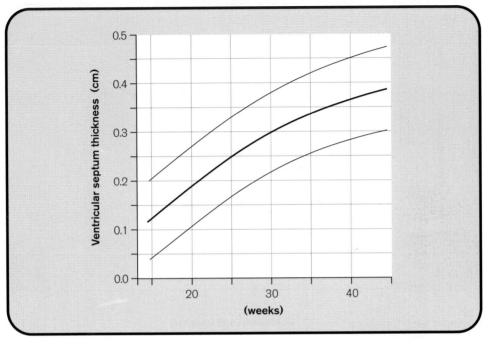

Figure 70 Thickness of the interventricular septum (regression line and 95% CI) from a study with cross-sectional and longitudinal data ($n=100$ observations). Subjects were healthy and had their menstrual dates confirmed by ultrasound measurements; they subsequently all delivered at term. The interventricular septal thickness was measured in the four-chamber view of the fetal heart, just below the atrioventricular valves. *Data source:* ref. 143, with permission, Excerpta Medica, Inc.

Comment: Thickness of the right or left ventricular wall is very similar to that of the interventricular septum.

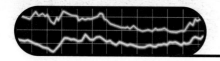

Ascending aorta and pulmonary artery diameter

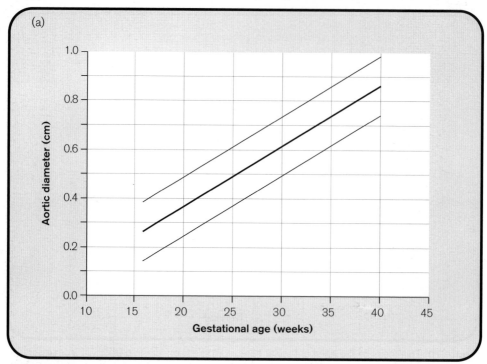

Figure 71 Diameter of (a) the ascending aorta.

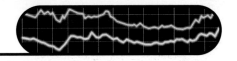

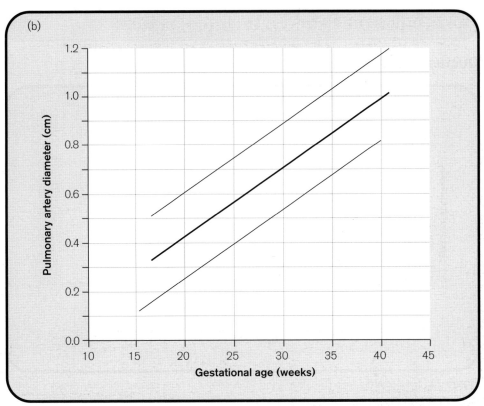

Figure 71 Diameter of (b) the main pulmonary artery (regression line and 95% prediction interval) from a cross-sectional study of 117 fetuses between 16 and 41 weeks' gestation, as described in Figure 69. The aorta was measured in a long-axis view of the heart, found by moving cephalad from the four-chamber view. Measurements were made between intimal surfaces when the aorta had been aligned perpendicular to the ultrasound beam, at a level just above the sinuses of Valsalva. The main pulmonary artery was measured in a long-axis view, aligning its vessel walls perpendicular to the ultrasound beam. *Data source:* ref. 142, with permission, Excerpta Medica Inc.

Comment: The pulmonary artery diameter is slightly larger than the aorta during intrauterine life. It may not be possible to obtain good views of these vessels in the planes described. However, in other studies where measurements have been made in different scan planes, values obtained have been similar.[143]

CARDIOVASCULAR DOPPLER INDICES

Ductus venosus

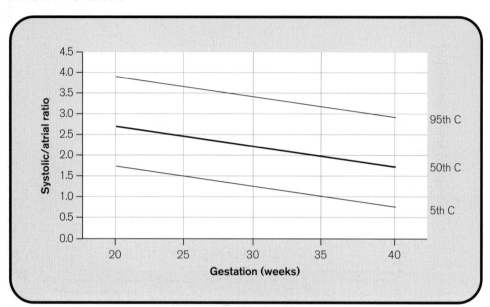

Figure 72 Systolic:atrial ratio (5th, 50th, and 95th centiles) from ductus venosus Doppler flow velocity waveforms. These were recorded in a cross-sectional study of 164 appropriate-for-gestational age fetuses at 16–42 weeks' gestation, who did not have structural or chromosomal abnormalities. Velocity waveforms were recorded from the ductus venosus at its origin from the umbilical vein as visualized in a transverse section of the fetal abdomen with a color and pulsed-Doppler machine. The angle of insonation of the vessel was kept low; any recordings where this angle exceeded 20° were rejected. The ductus venosus waveforms were recognized by their characteristic biphasic pattern. The ratio between peak systolic velocity and that occurring during atrial contraction (the nadir of the waveform) was calculated. *Data source:* ref. 144, with permission from Elsevier Science.

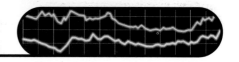

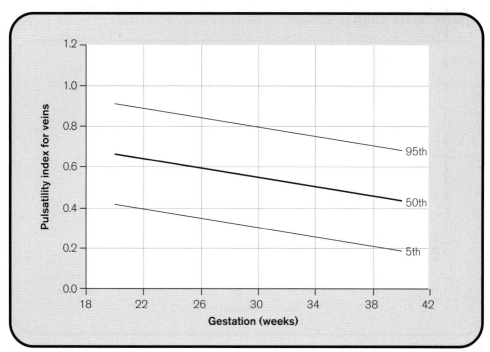

Figure 73 Pulsatility index for veins (PIV) from the ductus venosus (5th, 50th, and 95th centiles) from a cross-sectional study of 143 women with singleton pregnancies at 20–40 weeks' gestation. All fetuses were anatomically normal. Gestational age was calculated from menstrual history, confirmed by fetal measurements made at 20 weeks' amenorrhoea. At the time of study, fetuses had head and abdominal circumference measurements within the 90% CI for gestational age; and also normal movements, amniotic fluid volume, and an umbilical artery Doppler pulsatility index. All measurements were made in the absence of fetal breathing movements. Flow velocity waveforms were recorded from the ductus venosus, visualized in an oblique transverse plane through the upper abdomen or a mid-sagittal longitudinal plane. Good signals were obtained from 134 of the cases. PIV was calculated as (peak systolic velocity–minimum atrial velocity)/(time-averaged maximum velocity). *Data source:* ref. 145, with permission, Blackwell Science Limited.

Comment: Color-flow mapping Doppler equipment is necessary for the correct identification of the ductus venosus; waveforms from the intrahepatic portion of the umbilical vein and the inferior vena cava are different. The declining systolic:atrial ratio is interpreted as indicating a relative increase in blood flow during end diastole, i.e. improved cardiac filling.

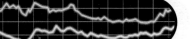

Inferior vena cava

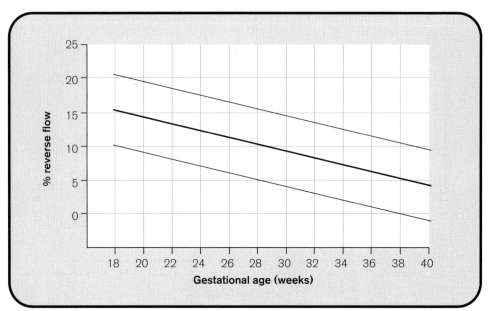

Figure 74 Percentage of reverse flow from the inferior vena cava (mean and linear regression of 95th CI) from a cross-sectional study of 118 appropriate-for-gestational-age fetuses of 18–40 weeks' gestation. All pregnancies were singleton, dated by certain last menstrual period and early second trimester ultrasonography. All fetuses were structurally normal and appropriate size for gestation at time of study. Flow velocity waveforms were recorded using color and pulsed-Doppler equipment from the inferior vena cava, identified in a sagittal view of the fetal trunk between the entrance of the renal vein and the ductus venosus. Measurements were made in the absence of fetal body or breathing movements. Three components of the waveform were identified: systolic peak (S), diastolic wave (D), and reverse flow during atrial contraction (A). The percentage of reverse flow was calculated as the percentage of the time–velocity integral during the A-wave, with respect to the total forward time velocity integral (S + D). *Data source:* ref. 146, with permission.

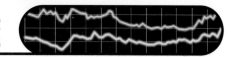

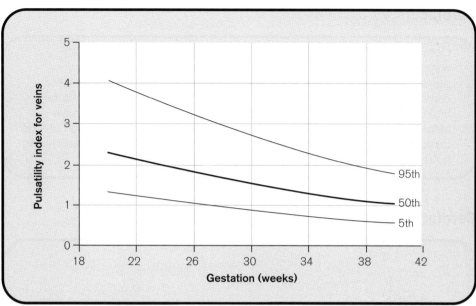

Figure 75 PIV from the inferior vena cava (5th, 50th, and 95th centiles) from the cross-sectional study of 143 women described in Figure 73. Flow velocity waveforms were recorded from the inferior vena cava in a longitudinal section of the fetal abdomen, with the sample volume placed in the portion between the renal and hepatic veins. Clear signals were obtained from 127 fetuses. PIV was calculated as (peak systolic velocity–minimum atrial velocity)/(time-averaged maximum velocity). *Data source:* ref. 145, with permission, Blackwell Science Limited.

Comment: Flow velocity waveforms in the inferior vena cava are characteristically triphasic, with reverse velocities during atrial contraction. There is a significant decrease in these reverse velocities with advancing gestation. This is attributed to a decrease in the pressure gradient between the right atrium and right ventricle at end diastole, due to improved ventricular compliance and reduced end-diastolic pressure. Right ventricular afterload declines with decreasing placental resistance, contributing to the reduction in end-diastolic pressure. In studies where Doppler waveforms have been recorded from the inferior vena cava and ductus venosus in growth-retarded fetuses prior to cordocentesis, fetal hypoxemia and acidemia have been found to be associated with more reverse flow and more pulsatile waveforms.[147,148]

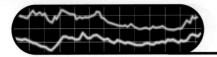

PHYSIOLOGY

Cardiac

> **Comment:** Normal ranges have been defined for Doppler flow velocity waveform indices derived from across the *mitral*, *tricuspid*, *aortic*, and *pulmonary* valves.[145,149,150] These have potential use in the assessment of cardiac function in growth-restricted fetuses and in fetuses with structural heart defects. Waveforms from the *ductus arteriosus* show considerable individual variability,[151] and do not appear to be useful in the detection of fetal compromise. Waveforms from *peripheral pulmonary arteries* show decreasing pulsatility with advancing gestation in healthy fetuses.[152]

Cardiac output

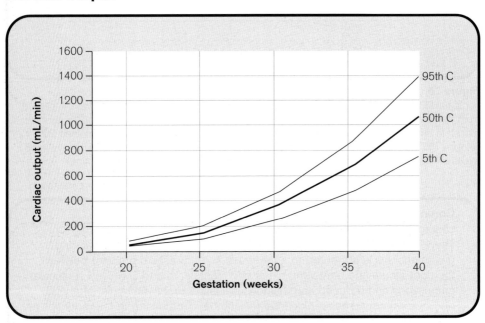

Figure 76 (a) Left cardiac output (LCO).

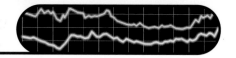

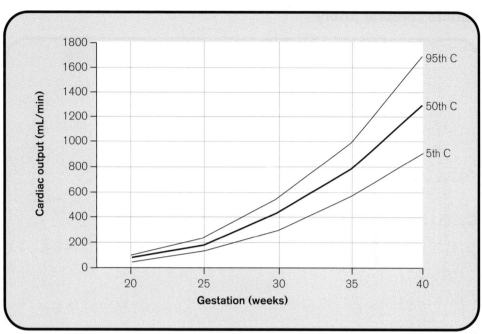

Figure 76 (b) Right cardiac output (RCO) calculated at the level of the outflow tracts (5th, 50th, and 95th centiles) from a longitudinal study of 26 healthy, singleton fetuses studied at weekly intervals. Velocity waveforms were recorded from the ascending aorta and pulmonary artery with the flow parallel to the Doppler beam; any recordings obtained with the beam angle greater than 20° were rejected. Valve diameter measurements were made from video tape images; valve areas were calculated by assuming a circular cross-section. *Data source:* ref. 149, with permission.

Comment: Cardiac output rises progressively with gestation, RCO being slightly higher than LCO (RCO/LCO ratio approximately 1.3). Peak flow velocity at both aortic and pulmonary valves rises with gestation. This is attributed to progressive improvement in cardiac contractility, reduction in afterload, and increase in preload.[149] Calculations of volume flow like these in fetal vessels are prone to high coefficients of variation as any error in the measurement of diameter (e.g. valve ring diameter) is further magnified as cross-sectional area is computed.

Middle cerebral artery

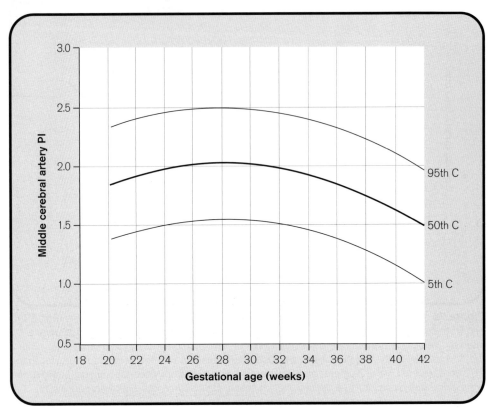

Figure 77 Pulsatility index from the middle cerebral artery (5th, 50th, and 95th centiles), from a cross-sectional study of 1556 fetuses at a gestational age of 20–42 weeks. All were singletons, and gestational age had been confirmed by early ultrasound measurement of CRL. Color flow imaging was used to identify the fetal middle cerebral artery, and waveforms were recorded at a low angle of insonation. Good signals were obtained from 1467 fetuses. The pulsatility index was calculated as (maximum systolic velocity − diastolic velocity)/(mean velocity). *Data source:* ref. 153, with permission.

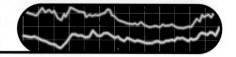

CARDIOVASCULAR DOPPLER INDICES

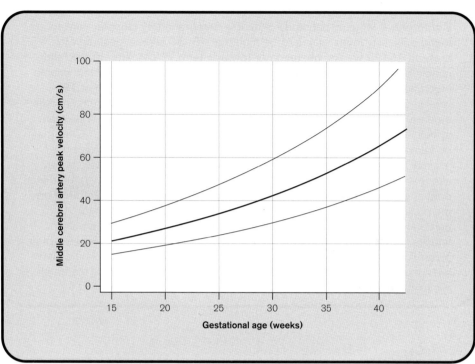

Figure 78 Peak velocity from the middle cerebral artery (mean and 95% prediction intervals) from a cross-sectional study of 135 normal fetuses between 15 and 42 weeks' gestation. The middle cerebral artery was identified in an axial section of the fetal brain, and insonated at a low angle. The highest point on the waveform (peak systolic velocity) was measured. *Data source:* ref. 154, with permission, Blackwell Science Limited.

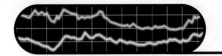

Comment: A longitudinal study of middle cerebral artery Doppler waveforms found pulsatility index values to be higher at 25–30 weeks' gestation than those at 15–20 weeks' gestation or towards term.[155] Diameter of the fetal middle cerebral artery increases with gestational age; the calculated volume blood flow in the artery increased in one study[156] from 23 ml/min at 19 weeks' gestation to 133 ml/min at term. Doppler waveforms from the middle cerebral artery may also be quantified using the resistance index (maximum systolic velocity – minimum diastolic velocity)/(systolic velocity).[157] Care must be taken when recording middle cerebral artery waveforms only to apply minimal pressure to the maternal abdomen, as fetal skull compression may alter middle cerebral artery flow.[158] Different signals are obtained in the distal portion of the middle cerebral artery, so most studies have concentrated on the proximal portion, close to the circle of Willis.[159] Changes in middle cerebral artery Doppler waveforms have been noted in growth-restricted fetuses, suggesting redistribution of the fetal cardiac output to preserve brain blood flow.[155,158,159] High middle cerebral artery peak systolic velocities have been associated with fetal anemia in pregnancies complicated by maternal alloimmunization.[154]

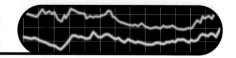

Descending aorta

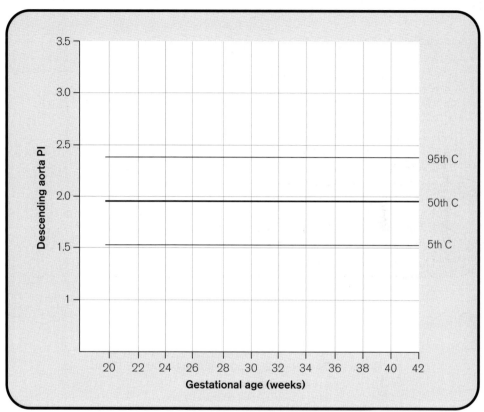

Figure 79 Descending aorta pulsatility index (5th, 50th, and 95th centiles) from a cross-sectional study of 1556 healthy pregnancies between 20 and 42 weeks' gestation. All were singletons, and gestational age had been confirmed by early ultrasound measurement of CRL. Recordings from the thoracic portion of the descending aorta were made in the absence of fetal body or breathing movements. Satisfactory recordings were obtained in 1398 fetuses. The pulsatility index was calculated as (systolic velocity − diastolic velocity)/(mean velocity). *Data source:* ref. 153, with permission.

Comment: There was no significant change with gestation in the aortic pulsatility index, unlike other fetal vessels.

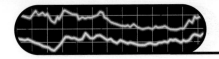

Umbilical artery

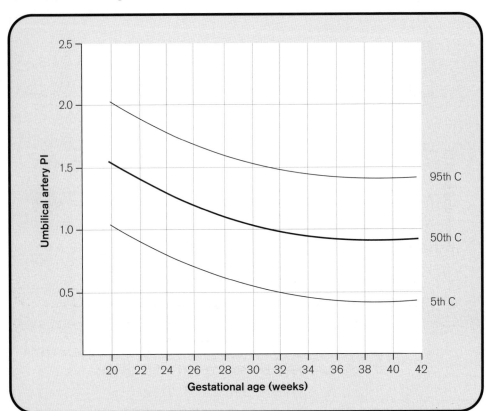

Figure 80 Umbilical artery pulsatility index (5th, 50th, and 95th centiles) from a cross-sectional study of 1556 healthy pregnancies between 20 and 42 weeks' gestation. All were singletons, and gestational age had been confirmed by early ultrasound measurement of CRL. Recordings from the umbilical artery were made in the absence of fetal body or breathing movements. The pulsatility index was calculated as (systolic velocity − diastolic velocity) (mean velocity). *Data source*: ref. 153, with permission.

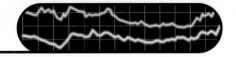

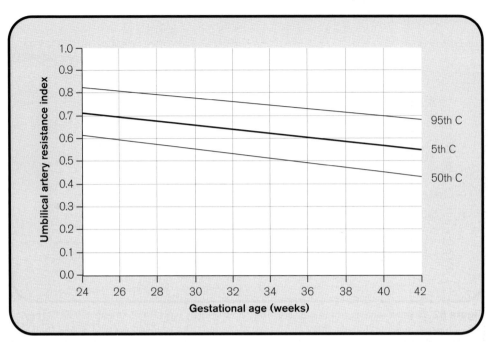

Figure 81 Umbilical artery resistance index (5th, 50th, and 95th centiles) from a cross-sectional study of 1675 pregnancies at 24–42 weeks' gestation. Each fetus only contributed one measurement to the study. Signals were recorded from a free-floating loop in the middle of the umbilical cord. *Data source*: ref. 157, with permission, Blackwell Science Limited.

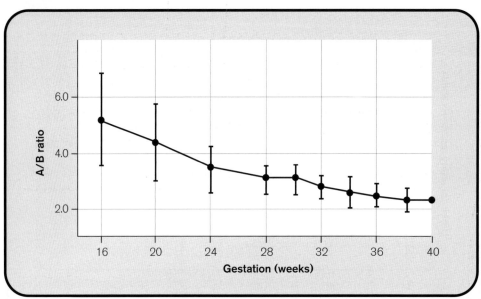

Figure 82 Doppler indices from umbilical artery flow velocity waveforms (mean ± 2 SD). They were obtained in a longitudinal study of 15 normal pregnancies scanned every 2 weeks from 24–28 weeks' gestation to delivery, eight of whom had been recruited at 16 weeks' gestation and also scanned every 4 weeks through the second trimester. In all subjects, gestational age had been confirmed by ultrasound scanning at 16 weeks' gestation. A range-gated pulsed Doppler beam was guided from the ultrasound image to insonate the umbilical artery. *A/B* ratio was calculated (where *A* is the maximum systolic frequency, *B* is the maximum diastolic frequency, as measured from the Doppler shift waveforms). *Data source*: ref. 160, with permission.

Comment (Figs 80–82): After 16 weeks' gestation there is forward flow in umbilical arteries throughout the cardiac cycle, as evidenced by positive Doppler shift frequencies even at the end of diastole. Declining values of the resistance index, pulsatility index, and *A/B* ratio with gestation are interpreted as indicating decreasing resistance in the placental circulation.

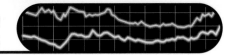

Fetal–placental Doppler ratios

Comment: Various ratios have been suggested comparing fetal cerebral flow velocity waveforms with those from the umbilical artery or aorta. They may be useful in detection of alteration in fetal cardiac output distribution, e.g. in response to fetal hypoxemia ('brain sparing' effect). The *placentocerebral ratio*[157] is (resistance indices from umbilical artery)/(middle cerebral artery); the *cerebroplacental ratio*[161] is (resistance indices from middle cerebral artery)/(umbilical artery); the *UA/MCA ratio*[153] is (pulsatility indices from umbilical artery)/(middle cerebral artery); and the *DA/MCA ratio*[153] is (pulsatility indices from descending thoracic aorta)/(middle cerebral artery).

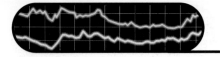

PHYSIOLOGY

CARDIOVASCULAR AND BEHAVIORAL PARAMETERS

Umbilical venous pressure (UVP)

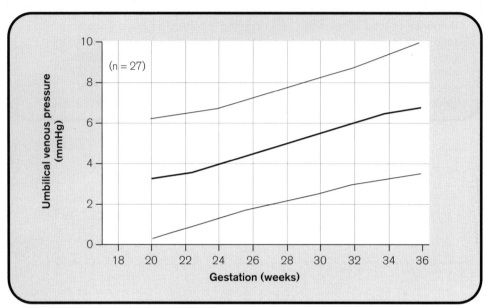

Figure 83 UVP (mean and 95% CI) from 27 fetuses referred for assessment of possible intrauterine infection or hemolysis, but subsequently shown to be unaffected. They all underwent cordocentesis, and after the necessary blood samples had been obtained the needle was connected to a pressure transducer. The transducer was placed at the level of the fetal heart, and the pressure read at its nadir. The needle was confirmed to be in the umbilical vein by the non-pulsatile pressure tracing obtained and by observing the direction of flow of injected saline. As the needle was withdrawn, the amniotic cavity pressure was recorded. UVP was calculated by subtracting amniotic pressure from the measured umbilical venous pressure. *Data source*: ref. 162, with permission, the American College of Obstetricians and Gynecologists.

Comment: UVP rises with advancing gestation, but remains within a narrow range. Values above the CI are associated with cardiac failure.[163]

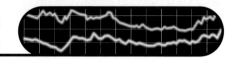
Mean umbilical arterial pressure (MAP)

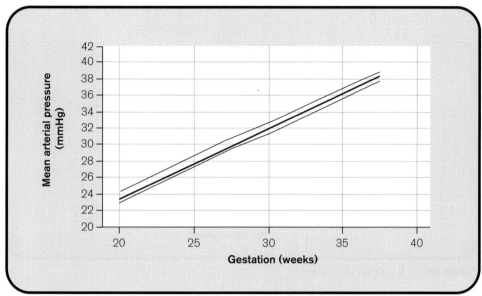

Figure 84 MAP (mean and 95% CI) from 30 normal fetuses. They had been referred for assessment of possible infection or hemolysis but were found to be unaffected. The methodology was identical to that outlined in Figure 66. It was apparent that the needle tip was in an umbilical artery rather than vein (due to a pulsatile pressure signal). *Data source:* ref. 164, with permission.

Comment: The normal range of arterial pressure in the fetus is very narrow (much more so than for umbilical venous pressure). Arterial pressure rises as gestational age increases.

Fetal heart rate (FHR)

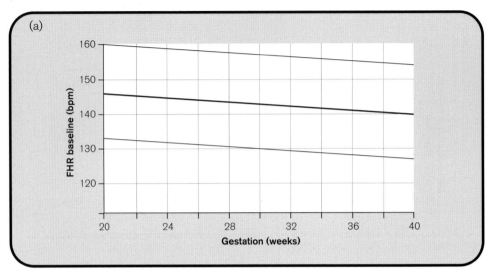

Figure 85 (a) Baseline heart rate.

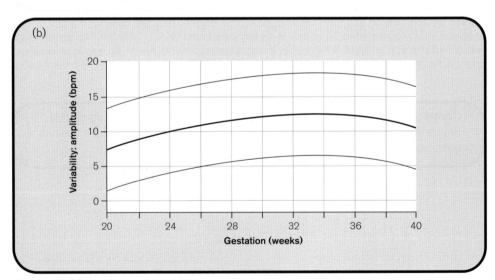

Figure 85 (b) Amplitude of variability.

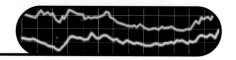

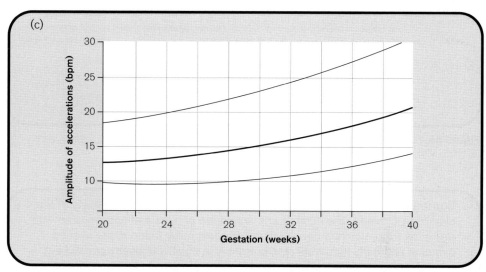

Figure 85 (c) Amplitude of accelerations.

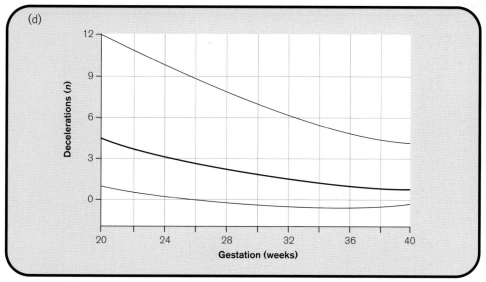

Figure 85 (d) Number of decelerations.

Figure 85 FHR parameters (mean and 95% CI) from a cross-sectional study of 119 pregnancies between 20 and 39 weeks' gestation who had been referred for prenatal diagnosis by cordocentesis. In all these cases, fetal blood gases, hemoglobin, and karyotype were subsequently shown to be normal; none had hydrops fetalis or any cardiac defect. FHR monitoring was performed immediately before cordocentesis for a period of 30 min. The traces were examined for FHR baseline, variability, accelerations, and decelerations. *Data source:* ref. 165, with permission from S Karger AG, Basel.

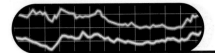

- At least two accelerations (>15 beats for >15 s) in 20 min, baseline heart rate 110–150 bpm, baseline variability 5–25 bpm, absence of decelerations.

- Sporadic decelerations amplitude <40 bpm are acceptable if duration <15 s, or <30 s following an acceleration.

- When there is moderate tachycardia (150–170 bpm) or brachycardia (100–110 bpm) a reactive trace is reassuring of good health.

Figure 86 Features of a normal antepartum cardiotocogram (non-stress test). *Data source: ref. 166, with permission.*

Comment: Baseline FHR decreases with gestation, but the variability of the baseline increases. The number and amplitude of accelerations increase with gestation. Spontaneous decelerations are commonly found in the second trimester and early third trimester, but rarely in healthy fetuses approaching term. Definitions of the features of normal and abnormal cardiotocograms are available.[167] During labor, criteria for the interpretation of FHR traces alter (see Fig. 104).

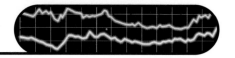

Biophysical profile score (BPS)

Fetal variable	Normal behavior (score = 2)	Abnormal behavior (score = 0)
Fetal breathing movements	More than 1 episode of 30 s duration, intermittent within a 30 min overall period. Hiccups count. (Not continuous throughout the observation time)	Repetitive or continuous breathing without cessation. Completely absent breathing or no sustained episodes
Gross body/limb movements	Three or more discrete body/limb movements in a 30 min period. Continuous active movement episodes are considered as a single movement. Also included are fine motor movements, positional adjustments and so on.	Two or fewer body/limb movements in a 30 min observation period
Fetal tone and posture	Demonstration of active extension with rapid return of flexion of fetal limbs, brisk repositioning/trunk rotation. Opening and closing of hand, mouth, kicking, etc.	Only low-velocity movements, incomplete return to flexion, flaccid extremity positions; abnormal fetal posture. Includes score = 0 when FM absent
Fetal heart rate reactivity	Greater than 2 significant accelerations associated with maternally palpated fetal movement during a 20 min cardiotocogram. (Accelerations graded for gestation: 10 beats/min for 10 s before 26 weeks; 15 beats/min for 15 s after 26 weeks; 20 beats/min for 20 s at term)	Fetal movement and accelerations not coupled. Insufficient accelerations, absent accelerations, or decelerative trace. Mean variation <20 on numerical analysis of CTG
Amniotic fluid volume evaluation	One pocket of >3 cm without umbilical cord loops. More than 1 pocket of >2 cm without cord loops. No elements of subjectively reduced amniotic volume.	No cord-free pocket >2 cm, or elements of subjectively reduced amniotic fluid volume definite

Figure 87 Scoring system for five fetal biophysical variables (breathing movements, gross body/limb movements, tone/posture, heart rate reactivity, and amniotic fluid volume) developed for the assessment of patients with high-risk pregnancies. This scoring system was evaluated in 216 patients who were studied in the week prior to delivery and whose eventual pregnancy outcome was documented. No perinatal deaths occurred in this study when all five variables were present at the time of examination with ultrasound and cardiotocography. Low scores (≤6 out of 10) were associated with increased incidence of adverse outcomes (fetal distress in labor, Apgar scores ≤7 at 5 min of age, perinatal death). *Data source*: ref. 168, with permission.

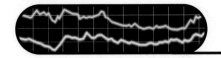

Comment: Various means of monitoring fetal well-being antenataly have been proposed (cardiotocography, observation of fetal breathing patterns, measurement of amniotic fluid volume); however, scoring systems which take into consideration a combination of behavioral parameters are superior in their ability to detect a compromised fetus and hence to allow its early delivery.[169] This has led to improvement in perinatal mortality rates, even in a high-risk group of pregnant women.[169] It must be borne in mind that fetal behavior is periodic and affected by external factors (e.g. maternal ingestion of stimulant or depressant drugs, maternal hypo- or hyperglycemia) and by structural or genetic abnormalities of the fetus. Fetal behavior abruptly changes from a quiescent to an active pattern and *vice versa*, thus ultrasound observation may need to be extended for 30 or 40 min to confirm absence of fetal movements or breathing; most BPS studies are completed in less than 10 min.[168] Acute disasters may occur which invalidate the predictive accuracy of the BPS (e.g. abruptio placentae, diabetic ketoacidosis, eclampsia).

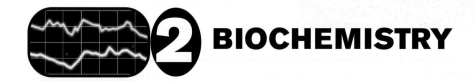 **2 BIOCHEMISTRY**

PROTEINS

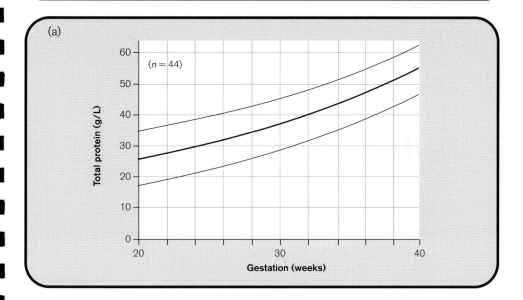

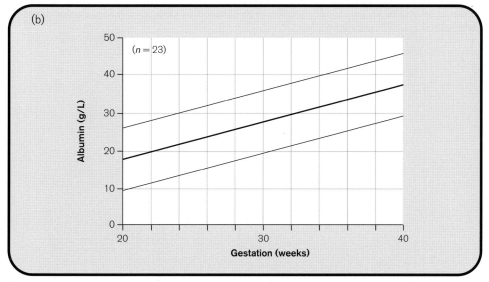

Figure 88 Total protein and albumin concentrations (regression curve and 95% CI) from a cross-sectional study of 45 fetuses, subsequently shown to be normal at birth. Blood samples were obtained by ultrasound-guided cordocentesis. *Data source*: ref. 170, with permission.

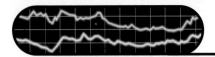

RENAL FUNCTION TESTS, LIVER FUNCTION TESTS AND GLUCOSE

	SI units (mean ± SD)	Traditional units (mean ± SD)
Glucose	4.3 ± 0.6 mmol/L	77 ± 11 mg/dl
Cholesterol	1.5 ± 0.3 mmol/L	59 ± 11 mg/dl
Uric acid	179 ± 39 µmol/L	2.8 ± 0.6 mg/dl
Triglycerides	4.5 ± 1.1 mmol/L	40 ± 10 mg/dl
Total bilirubin	26.3 ± 5.8 µmol/L	1.5 ± 0.3 mg/dl
Alkaline phosphatase	260 ± 65 IU/L	
Gamma glutamyl transferase	60 ± 34 IU/L	
Asparate transaminase	17 ± 6.5 IU/L	
Creatinine	1.8 ± 0.3 µmol/L	0.02 ± 0.003 mg/dl
Calcium	2.3 ± 0.2 mmol/L	9.2 ± 0.8 mg/dl

Figure 89 Glucose, calcium, liver function, and renal function tests (mean ± SD) from a cross-sectional study of 78 fetuses of gestational age 20–26 weeks; all fetuses were subsequently shown to be healthy at birth. Blood samples were obtained by ultrasound-guided cordocentesis. *Data source*: ref. 171, with permission.

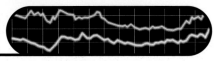

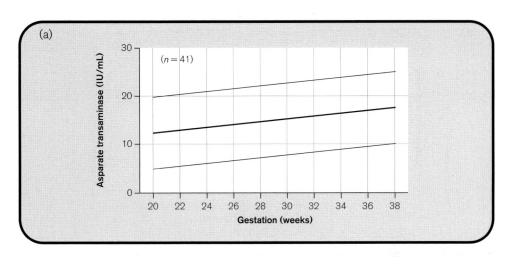

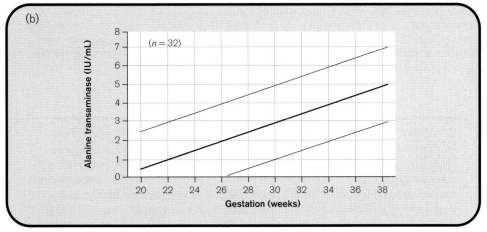

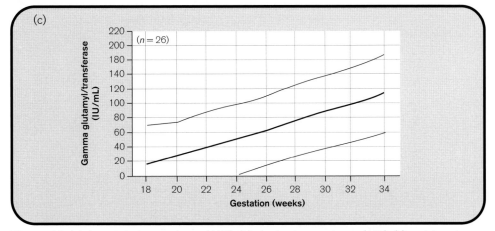

Figure 90 (a) Aspartate transaminase (AST), (b) alanine transaminase (ALT), (c) γ-glutamyl transferase (GGT).

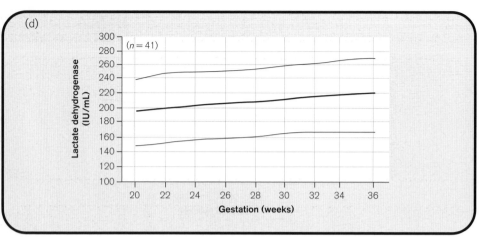

Figure 90 (d) lactate dehydrogenase (LDH) concentrations (regression line and 95% CI) from a cross-sectional study of 80 fetuses referred for assessment of possible intrauterine infection or hemolysis, but subsequently shown to be unaffected. They underwent cordocentesis, and blood samples were obtained for liver enzyme assays (the numbers of assays performed for each enzyme are stated on individual graphs). *Data source:* ref. 162, with permission, the American College of Obstetricians and Gynecologists.

Comment (Figs 88–90): Plasma total protein and albumin concentrations increase significantly with gestational age.[170] Little information is available regarding many of the other biochemical variables: triglyceride levels fall with advancing gestation,[171] bilirubin levels rise,[172] and liver enzyme concentrations (apart from LDH) rise.[162] Fetal concentrations of bilirubin are higher, and those of triglyceride and cholesterol lower, than in maternal serum.[171] Fetal plasma insulin levels rise with gestation.[173]

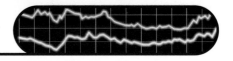

URINARY BIOCHEMISTRY

(a)	16 weeks	33 weeks
Phosphate (mmol/L)	0.91	0.10
Creatinine (µmol/L)	99.9	172.9
(mean values)		

(b)	Mean value	95% confidence intervals (CI)
Potassium (mmol/L)	3.0	0–6.1
Calcium (mmol/L)	0.21	0.04–1.2
Urea (µmol/L)	7.9	2.6–13.1

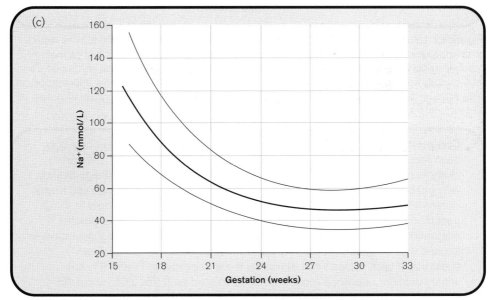

Figure 91 Urinary electrolyte levels from a study of 26 women between 16 and 33 weeks' gestation, with normal amniotic fluid volume and normal fetal anatomy: (a) phosphate and creatinine; (b) potassium, calcium, and urea; and (c) sodium (mean and 95% CI where computed). Seventeen of the women had pregnancies complicated by rhesus alloimmunization; in these the fetal bladder was emptied prior to intraperitoneal blood transfusion. The other women had aspiration of the fetal bladder prior to therapeutic termination of pregnancy. *Data source:* ref. 174, with permission.

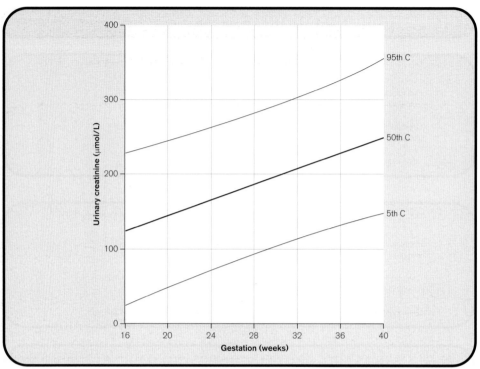

Figure 92 Urinary creatinine (5th, 50th, and 95th centiles) from a study of 20 fetuses with obstructive uropathy who had no features of renal dysplasia and subsequently had normal postnatal renal function. Ultrasound-guided needle aspiration of fetal urine was performed. The fetal bladder was aspirated when there was distention of the bladder and similar appearances of both kidneys; the renal pelvis was aspirated when there was unilateral pelvicalyceal dilatation. In all cases, fetal karyotype was normal. *Data source:* ref. 175, with permission.

Comment (Figs 91 and 92): Fetal urinary biochemistry has previously only been studied indirectly from examination of the amniotic fluid.[140] This direct study found that urinary sodium and phosphate levels decreased significantly with gestational age over the period studied (16–33 weeks); creatinine levels increased. Urinary potassium, calcium, and urea levels did not show gestational changes. The pattern of electrolyte changes suggests parallel maturation of both glomerular and tubular function with advancing gestation. In fetuses with obstructive uropathy but normal postnatal renal function,[175] sodium and urea values were similar to those reported in Figure 91, but urinary calcium reference ranges were calculated as 0.25, 0.95, and 1.65 mmol/L (5th, 50th, and 95th centiles). Various groups have suggested adverse prognostic urinary electrolyte values, *e.g.* sodium values over 100 mmol/L, creatinine over 150 μmol/L (1.7 mg/dl), calcium over 2 mmol/L (8 mg/dl), and osmolality over 200 mOsm/L, but these are not universally accepted.[176,177] It may be seen from the data presented here that a sodium concentration of over 100 mmol/L may be normal for fetuses of less than 20 weeks' gestation.

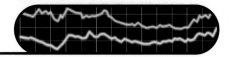

BLOOD GASES

Oxygen pressure (P_{O_2}), carbon dioxide pressure (P_{CO_2}), pH, base deficit

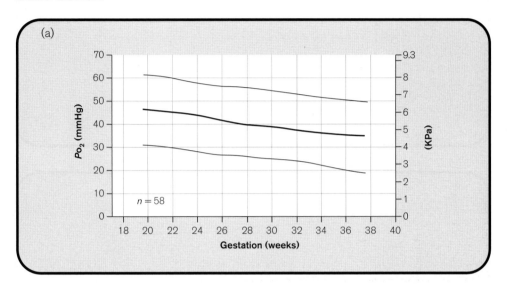

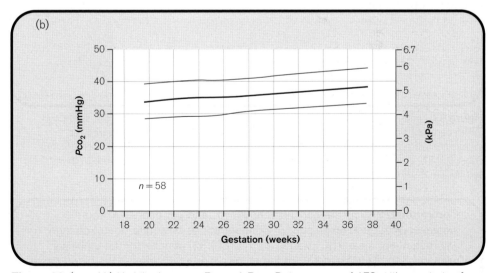

Figure 93 (a and b) Umbilical venous P_{O_2} and P_{CO_2}. Data source: ref 178, with permission from Elsevier Science.

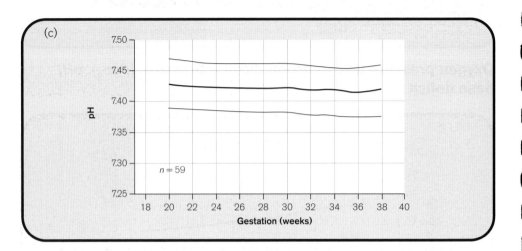

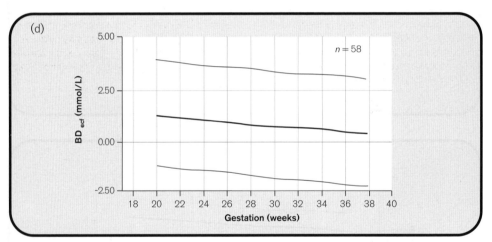

Figure 93 Umbilical venous pH, and base deficit of the extracellular fluid (2.5th, 50th, and 97.5th centiles) from a cross-sectional study of 59 fetuses who had been referred for assessment of possible intrauterine infection or hemolysis, but were found to be unaffected. Subsequently, all were healthy at birth and appropriately grown. *Data source:* ref. 178, with permission, Elsevier Science.

Comment: Umbilical arterial and venous Po_2 and pH decrease, and Pco_2 increases with gestational age.[179] Concentrations of lactate do not change with gestation; mean (SD) values are 0.99 (0.32) mmol/L for the umbilical vein and 0.92 (0.21) mmol/L for the umbilical artery.[179] Intervillous blood has a higher Po_2 and lower Pco_2, than, but similar pH and lactate concentrations to, umbilical venous blood.[180] The decrease in Po_2 in umbilical venous blood with advancing gestation is offset by increasing fetal hemoglobin concentration, such that the blood oxygen content remains constant; the mean umbilical venous oxygen content is 6.7 (0.6) mmol/L.[180]

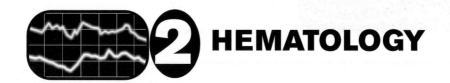

2 HEMATOLOGY

FULL BLOOD COUNT (FBC)

Gestational age (weeks)	WBC (10⁹/L)	PLT (10⁹/L)	RBC (10¹²/L)	Hb (g/dL)	MCV (fL)
18–23 ($n = 771$)	4.41 ± 1.2	241 ± 45	2.87 ± 0.2	11.7 ± 0.8	131.2 ± 7.3
24–29 ($n = 407$)	4.6 ± 1.3	267 ± 49	3.38 ± 0.32	12.8 ± 1.1	119.1 ± 5.6
30–35 ($n = 55$)	5.8 ± 1.6	265 ± 59	3.86 ± 0.43	14.1 ± 1.4	114.3 ± 7

Figure 94 Red cell count (RBC), white cell count (WBC), platelets (PLT), hemoglobin (Hb), and mean cell volume (MCV) from a cross-sectional study of 1233 normal fetuses between 18 and 36 weeks' gestation (mean ± SD). These were pregnancies referred for fetal blood sampling for prenatal diagnosis (mostly toxoplasmosis), but the fetuses were normal and subsequently shown to be healthy at birth. Fetal blood samples were taken by ultrasound-guided cordocentesis. *Data source:* ref. 171, with permission.

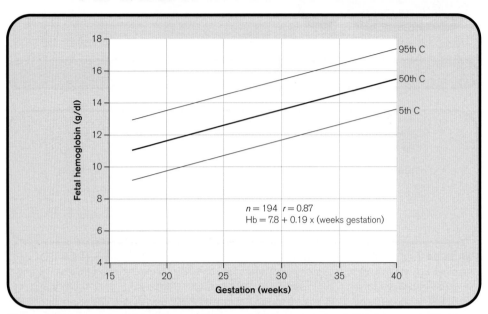

Figure 95 Hemoglobin (5th, 50th, and 95th centiles) from a study of 194 fetuses at 17–40 weeks' gestation. The fetuses were undergoing prenatal diagnosis but were found to be unaffected for the condition tested. *Data source*: ref. 181, with permission.

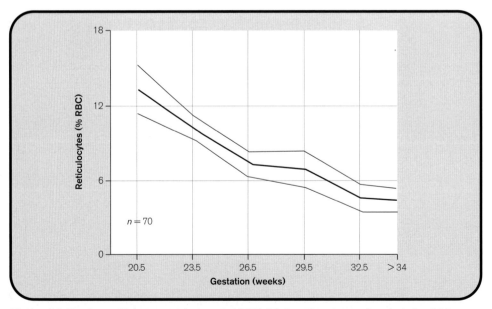

Figure 96 Fetal reticulocyte count (mean and 95% CI) from a cross-sectional study of 81 fetuses referred for prenatal diagnosis for a variety of indications, but subsequently shown to be unaffected. Ultrasound-guided cordocentesis was performed in order to obtain blood samples. *Data source*: ref. 182, with permission.

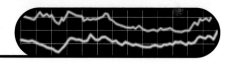

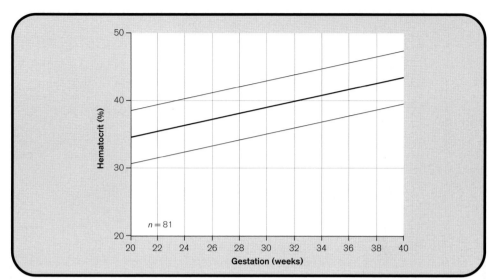

Figure 97 Hematocrit (regression line and 95% CI) from a cross-sectional study of 81 fetuses referred for prenatal diagnosis for a variety of indications, but subsequently shown to be unaffected. Ultrasound-guided cordocentesis was performed in order to obtain blood samples. *Data source:* ref. 182, with permission.

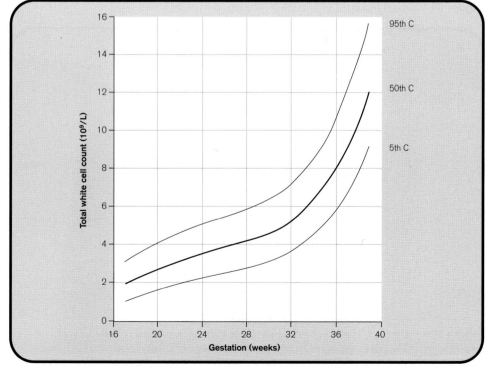

Figure 98 (a) Total white cell.

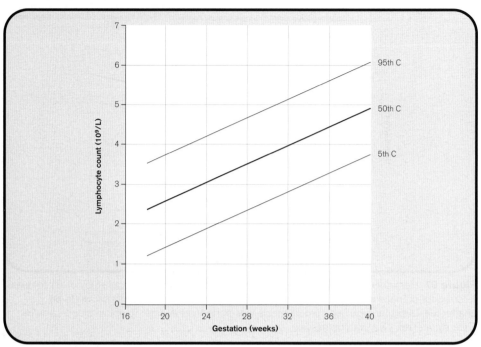

Figure 98 (b) lymphocyte.

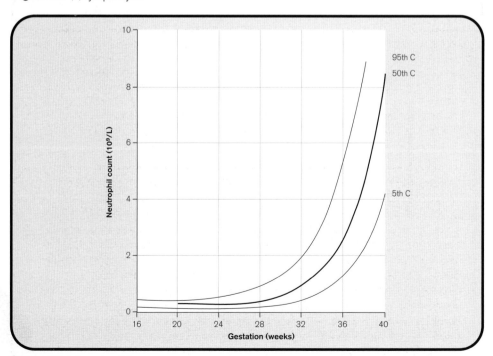

Figure 98 (c) neutrophil.

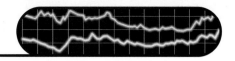

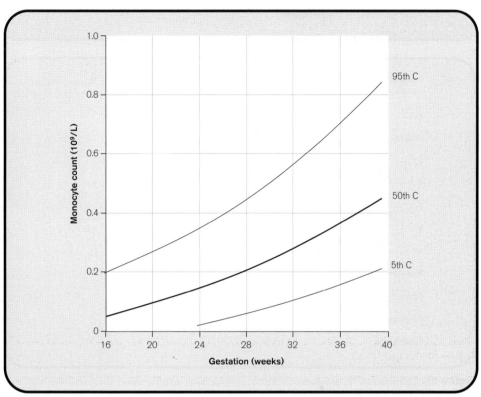

Figure 98 (d) monocyte counts (5th, 50th, and 95th centiles) from umbilical cord blood samples obtained at cordocentesis ($n = 316$) or elective cesarean delivery ($n = 11$) from fetuses between 18 and 40 weeks' gestation. Cordocentesis was performed for karyotyping, prenatal diagnosis, investigation of infection, or for blood grouping, but all fetuses included in this study were unaffected by the condition being investigated. The fetuses investigated at the time of elective cesarean delivery were all normal and appropriately grown; the indication for cesarean section was a breech presentation or a uterine scar. *Data source*: ref. 183, with permission.

Comment (Figs 94–98): The fetal red cell count and total hemoglobin increase linearly, the reticulocyte count decreases linearly, and the erythroblast count decreases exponentially with gestation.[181–183] The platelet count does not change.[171] Lymphocytes form the main population of white cells in the fetus until 37–38 weeks' gestation.[183] From 32 weeks' gestation onwards, neutrophils become more plentiful, and by term form approximately 60% of the total white cell count.[183] Natural killer cells are the main circulating white cell type in the first trimester of pregnancy.[183,184] Interferon-γ concentrations (5th–95th centiles) are high in the first trimester (0.4–3.1 U/mL), decreasing to 0.2–1.7 U/mL in the third trimester.[184] Fetal hemoglobin (Hb F) decreases with advancing gestation, from over 80% of the total hemoglobin in mid-pregnancy to approximately 70% by term.[171]

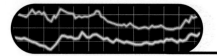

COAGULATION FACTORS

Coagulation factors	%	Inhibitors	%
VIIIC	40 ± 12	Fibronectin	40 ± 10
VIIIRAg	60 ± 13	Protein C	11 ± 3
VII	28 ± 5	α_2-Macroglobulin	18 ± 4
IX	9 ± 3	α_1-Antitrypsin	40 ± 4
V	47 ± 10	AT III	30 ± 3
II	12 ± 3	α_2-Antiplasmin	61 ± 6
XII	22 ± 3		
Prekallikrein	19 ± 2		
Fibrin-stabilizing factor	30 ± 5		
Fibrinogen	40 ± 15		
Plasminogen	24 ± 15		

Figure 99 Coagulation factors (percentage of normal adult values; mean ± 1 SD) from a cross-sectional study of 103 fetuses of 19–27 weeks' gestation, subsequently shown to be healthy. Blood samples were obtained by ultrasound-guided cordocentesis. *Data source*: ref. 171, with permission.

Comment: No changes in levels or activity of the various coagulation factors and their inhibitors were observed through the 8 weeks of gestation studied.

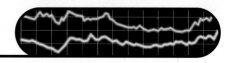

IRON METABOLISM

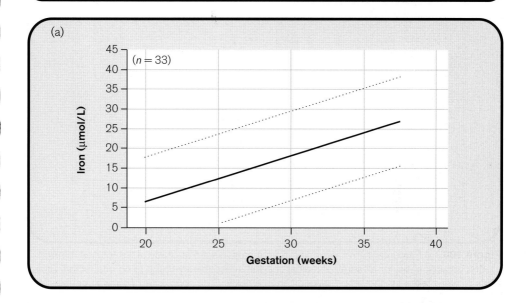

(a)

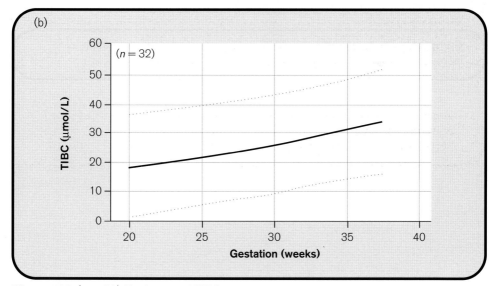

(b)

Figure 100 (a and b) Fetal iron and TIBC.

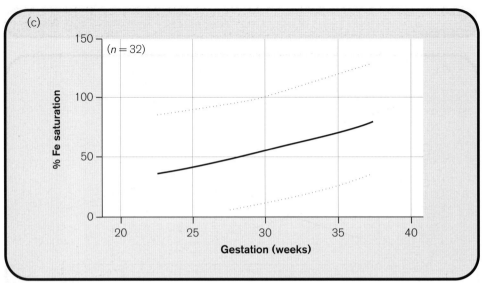

Figure 100 (c) Percentage iron saturation from a cross-sectional study of 33 fetuses referred for prenatal diagnosis for a variety of indications, but subsequently found to be unaffected. Blood samples were taken by ultrasound-guided cordocentesis. *Data source*: ref. 185, with permission.

Comment: The fetal iron level, TIBC, and percentage iron saturation all increase with advancing gestation.

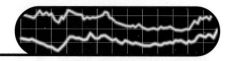

AMNIOTIC FLUID BILIRUBIN

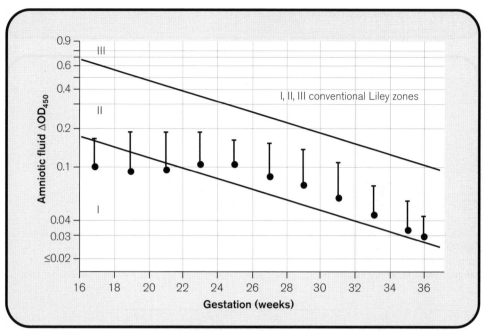

Figure 101 Amniotic fluid bilirubin ΔOD_{450} (mean $\pm$ 2 SD) from 475 samples of amniotic fluid obtained from pregnancies between 16 and 36 weeks' gestation not complicated by fetal hemolysis. Amniotic fluid samples taken at the time of fetoscopy or by amniocentesis were placed in darkened containers to protect against photodecomposition, and centrifuged to remove vernix and cellular debris. The bilirubin concentration was measured spectrophotometrically by the deviation in optical density of the amniotic fluid at a wavelength of 450 nm. *Data source*: ref. 186, with permission.

Comment: The normal range of liquor ΔOD_{450} does not change between the gestational ages of 16 and 25 weeks, but values fall during the third trimester and are widely scattered.

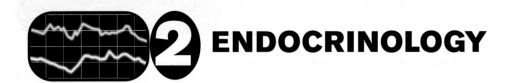

THYROID FUNCTION

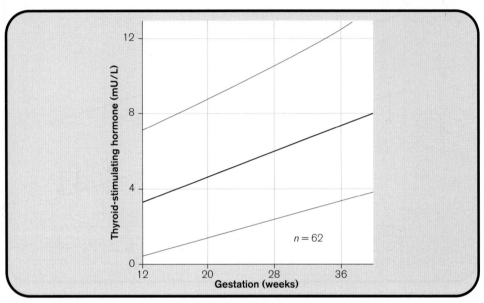

Figure 102 (a) Thyroid-stimulating hormone (TSH). Redrawn from ref 187.

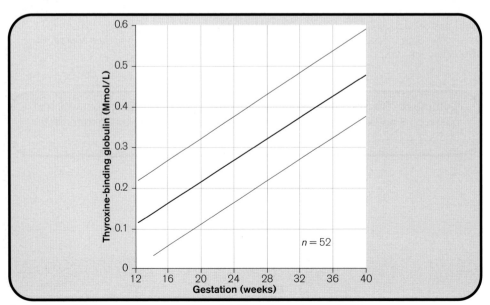

Figure 102 (b) Thyroxine-binding globulin (TBG). Redrawn from ref 187.

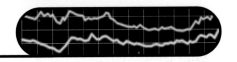

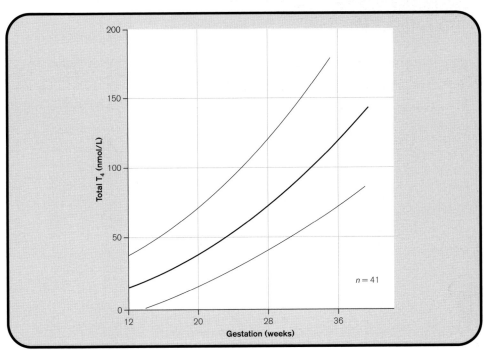

Figure 102 (c) Total T$_4$.

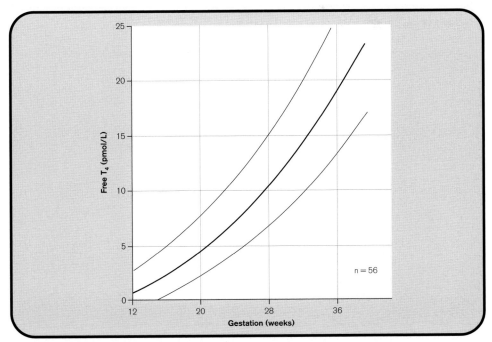

Figure 102 (d) Free T$_4$.

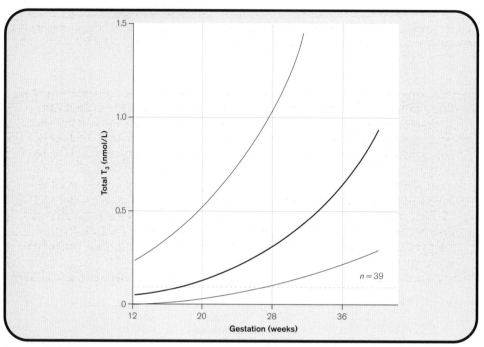

Figure 102 (e) Total T$_3$.

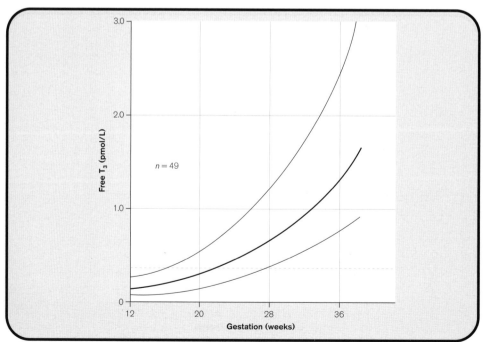

Figure 102 (f) Free T$_3$.

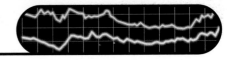

Figure 102 Thyroid function tests from a study of 62 women who underwent cordocentesis or cardiocentesis for prenatal diagnosis, and whose fetuses were subsequently shown to be normal (mean, 5th and 95th centiles). The dashed line is the lower limit of sensitivity of the assay. *Data source*: ref. 187, with permission.

Comment: No significant associations have been found between fetal and maternal thyroid hormones and TSH concentrations, suggesting that the fetal pituitary–thyroid axis is independent of that of its mother.[187] Fetal TSH levels are always higher than those in the mother. Free and total T_4 levels and those of TBG rise through pregnancy, and reach adult levels by 36 weeks' gestation; however, free and total T_3 levels are always substantially less than adult levels. The increase in fetal blood levels of TSH, thyroid hormones, and TBG during pregnancy indicates independent and autonomous maturation of the pituitary, thyroid, and liver respectively.[187] There does not appear to be feedback control of pituitary secretion of TSH by circulating thyroid hormones *in utero*.

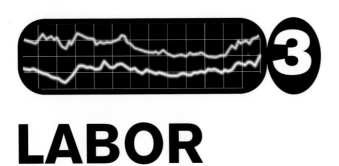

LABOR

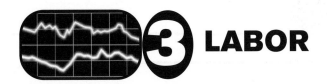

3 LABOR

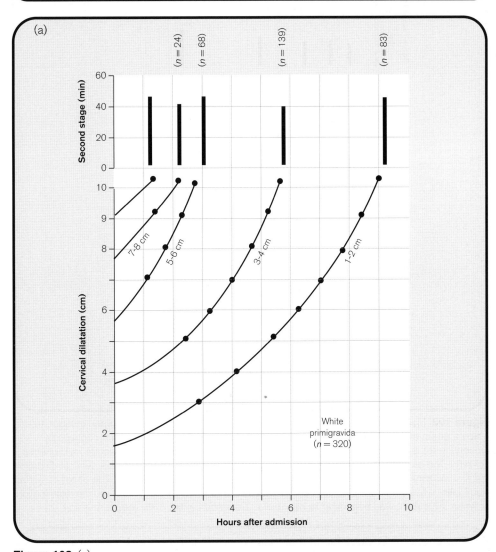

Figure 103 (a)

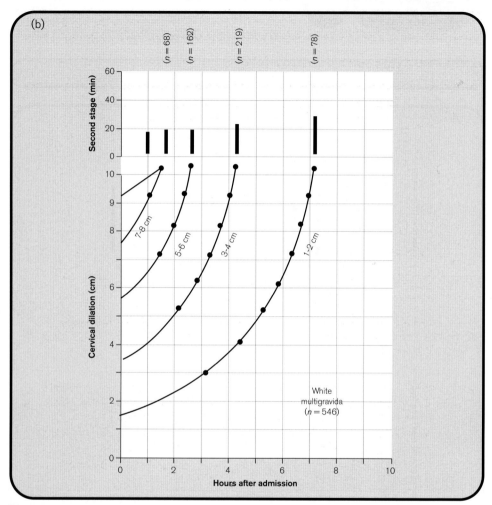

Figure 103 Mean cervimetric progress from a study of 3217 consecutive women in labor, from which a group of 1306 who had normal labor were identified (i.e. women with a cephalically presenting fetus, who did not have epidural block, receive oxytocic drugs, or require instrumental delivery). The progress of labor was followed by vaginal examination to establish cervical dilatation, the first examination being performed soon after admission to the labor suite. The onset of second stage labor was confirmed when full cervical dilatation was found at the time of routine examination, or when the patient was beginning to bear down. *Data source*: ref. 188, with permission.

Comment: This study found that mean cervimetric progress from 1 to 7 cm was faster in Caucasian multiparae than primiparae, but thereafter progress in the two groups was similar. No significant differences in the cervimetric progress of labor between women from different racial groups has been found.[188] The mean duration of the second stage of labor is approximately 42 min in primiparae and 17 min in multiparae,[188] although it is recognized that the precise onset of full cervical dilatation is difficult to establish.

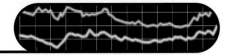

FHR PARAMETERS BY CARDIOTOCOGRAPHY

Admission test cardiotocography

Admission test CTG
- At least two accelerations (>15 beats for >15 s) in 20 minutes.
- Baseline heart rate 110–150 bpm.
- Baseline variability 5–25 bpm.
- Absence of decelerations.
- Moderate tachycardia/bradycardia and accelerations.

First stage intrapartum CTG
- At least two accelerations (>15 beats for >15 s) in 20 minutes.
- Baseline heart rate 110–150 bpm.
- Baseline variability 5–25 bpm.
- Early decelerations (in late first stage of labor).

Second stage intrapartum CTG
- Normal baseline heart rate, normal baseline variability and no decelerations, both periodic and scattered.
- Baseline heart rate 110–150 bpm and baseline variability 5–25 bpm or >25 bpm, with or without early and/or variable decelerations.

Figure 104 Features of the normal cardiotocogram (CTG) in labor. *Data source*: ref. 166, with permission, Elsevier Science.

Comment: Decelerations, which are abnormal if identified antepartum (see Fig. 86), are often encountered intrapartum. Early decelerations (i.e. synchronous with contractions) are common toward the end of the first stage of labor; during the second stage of labor both early and variable decelerations can be normal findings. Accelerations and normal baseline variability are important features of a healthy CTG.

UMBILICAL CORD BLOOD SAMPLING

Blood gases

		Umbilical artery	Umbilical vein
pH		7.06–7.36	7.14–7.45
P_{O_2}			
	(kPa)	1.3–5.5	1.7–6.0
	(mmHg)	9.8–41.2	12.3–45.0
P_{CO_2}			
	(kPa)	9.1–3.7	7.5–3.2
	(mmHg)	68.3–27.8	56.3–24.0
BD_{ecf}	(mmol/L)	15.3–0.5	12.6–0.7

Figure 105 Umbilical artery and vein blood gas values (pH, P_{O_2}, P_{CO_2}, extracellular base deficit) from a study lasting 2 years in a University hospital in The Netherlands, where cord blood samples were taken from all deliveries (95% CI). A piece of umbilical cord was isolated as soon as possible after delivery, and arterial and venous samples taken into two heparinized syringes. Samples were analyzed within 75 min of delivery by an automated blood gas machine. If the difference between pH values in the umbilical artery and vein was not at least 2 pH units, the arterial sample was rejected. Thus, 4667 arterial and 5151 venous pH samples were obtained. Smaller numbers of samples also had P_{O_2} and P_{CO_2} values measured. *Data source:* ref. 189, with permission.

Comment: There was a negatively skewed distribution of pH values overall. This data set was large enough to allow subanalysis. Values for pH were lower following cesarean section or breech delivery than after spontaneous vertex delivery (10th centiles for pH in these groups were 7.12, 7.11, and 7.15, respectively). Optimal cases (no problems antenatally or during labor, spontaneous labor, second stage less than 30 min, vertex presentation, normally grown infant in good condition at birth) had 10th centile pH values of 7.17. There were only small differences in pH between samples obtained from premature, mature, and postmature infants. Guidelines are available for optimal collection and analytical techniques.[178]

Lactate

Comment: Mean umbilical cord lactate values were reported as 1.87 mmol/L (SD 0.94 mmol/L) in a study of more than 3000 spontaneous vaginal deliveries.[190] Lower values were found after elective cesarean delivery (mean 1.44 mmol/L, SD 0.10 mmol/L, $n = 300$).

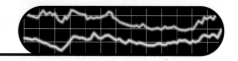

Full blood count

Analyte	25th centile	50th centile	75th centile
Red cell count ($\times 10^{12}$/L)	4.13	4.40	4.62
Hemoglobin (mmol/L)	9.5	10.0	10.7
(g/dl)	15.3	16.1	17.2
Hematocrit (%)	45.2	47.9	50.9
Mean cell volume (fl)	107.4	109.8	113.3
Mean cell hemoglobin (fmol)	2.2	2.3	2.4
(pg)	35.4	37.1	38.7
Reticulocyte count ($\times 10^9$/L)	145.8	170.0	192.6
Platelet count ($\times 10^9$/L)	237	270	321
Total white cell count ($\times 10^9$/L)	11.1	13.3	16.2
Neutrophil ($\times 10^9$/L)	5.4	7.4	8.8
Lymphocyte ($\times 10^9$/L)	3.3	3.8	5.1
Monocyte ($\times 10^9$/L)	1.2	1.6	2.3
Eosinophil ($\times 10^9$/L)	0.23	0.39	0.54
Basophil ($\times 10^9$/L)	0.04	0.06	0.09

Figure 106 Red cell count, hemoglobin, hematocrit, mean cell volume, mean cell hemoglobin, reticulocyte count, platelet count, and differential white cell count (25th, 50th and 75th centiles) from a study of 89 women who had been healthy during pregnancy and were non-smokers. All delivered after 34 weeks' gestation, and their infants were of normal birth weight and had an umbilical cord pH above 7.20. Umbilical venous samples were taken and analyzed within 3 h. *Data source:* ref. 191, with permission from Elsevier Science.

Comment: Infants of smokers were found in this study to have lower reticulocyte and neutrophil counts.[191] The reticulocyte counting was done by flow cytometry, which is more precise than manual counting. Full-term cord blood has more immature reticulocyte forms than does adult blood.[192] Another recent study found very similar blood count values,[193] and recommended that the lower limit for the normal hemoglobin level be designated as 12.5 g/dl for term newborns.

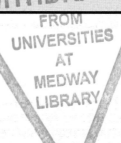

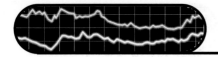

Biochemistry

Analyte	Cord arterial (n = 179)	Cord venous (n = 390)	Adult
Na⁺ (mmol/L)	135–143	135–143	136–146
K⁺ (mmol/L)	3.7–6.4	3.8–6.8	3.6–4.8
Cl⁻ (mmol/L)	102–111	102–112	96–110
Glucose (mmol/L)	2.3–6.7	2.9–7.4	4.4–6.1
Urea (mmol/L)	1.8–5.6	1.8–5.4	2.5–8.5
Creatinine (µmol/L)	45–96	51–97	65–125
Urate (µmol/L)	186–480	200–456	150–480
Phosphate (mmol/L)	1.23–2.14	1.31–2.18	0.80–1.60
Ca²⁺ (mmol/L)	2.16–2.94	2.32–2.99	2.10–2.60
Albumin (g/L)	26–40	30–41	35–48
Total protein (g/L)	43–67	46–68	60–80
Cholesterol (mmol/L)	0.8–2.5	0.9–2.5	<5.2
ALP (U/L)	77–285	87–303	36–135 (20–55 years) 37–160 (55–74 years) 50–200 (>75 years)
ALT (U/L)	4–24	4–27	5–40
AST (U/L)	16–63	17–59	10–30
CK (U/L)	71–475	82–528	10–180
LD (U/L)	206–580	201–494	90–230
CO₂ (mmol/L)	13–29	15–28	24–30
GGT (U/L)	20–302	27–339	8–50 (male) 6–50 (female)
Triglyceride (mmol/L)	0.10–1.04	0.13–0.97	0.55–1.7
Mg²⁺ (mmol/L)	0.49–0.80	0.50–0.79	0.6–1.0

ALP, alkaline phosphatase; ALT, alanine aminotransferase; AST, aspartate aminotransferase; LD, lactate dehydrogenase

Figure 107 Clinical chemistry analytes (95% CI) from umbilical arterial and venous blood, as compared to adult blood values. Samples were taken into heparinized tubes from the umbilical cords of 397 infants delivered between 37 and 41 weeks' gestation, before placental expulsion from the uterus. There were 310 vaginal deliveries and 87 cesarean deliveries. All babies included in the study had 5 min Apgar scores ≥ 8. Samples were stored at 4°C until analysis. Complete biochemistry profiles were obtained from 390 venous plasma and 179 arterial plasma samples. These were compared to the adult reference ranges from the institution (Ottawa Civic Hospital, Canada). *Data source:* ref. 194, with permission.

Comment: All cord blood chemistry values were found to be significantly different from adult values. There were no male:female differences identified. Cord creatine kinase concentrations were very high, although they were similar in infants after vaginal as cesarean delivery, suggesting that this did not relate to physical trauma.

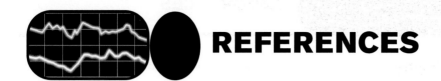

REFERENCES

REFERENCES

1. Dawes MG, Grudzinkas JG (1991) Patterns of maternal weight gain in pregnancy. Br J Obstet Gynaecol 98: 195–201. Blackwell Science Ltd.
2. National Academy of Sciences (1990) Nutrition during pregnancy. National Academy Press, Washington, DC.
3. Rosso P (1985) A new chart to monitor weight gain during pregnancy. Am J Clin Nutr 41: 644–652.
4. National Academy of Sciences (1989) Recommended dietary allowances, 10th edn. National Academy Press, Washington, DC.
5. MacGillivray I, Rose GA, Rowe B (1969) Blood pressure survey in pregnancy. Clin Sci 37: 395–407. Portland Press Limited.
6. Spatling L, Fallenstein F, Huch A, Huch R, Rooth G (1992) The variability of cardiopulmonary adaptation to pregnancy at rest and during exercise. Br J Obstet Gynaecol 99 (suppl 8). Blackwell Science Ltd.
7. Clapp JF III (1985) Maternal heart rate in pregnancy. Am J Obstet Gynecol 152: 659–660.
8. Clark SL, Cotton DB, Lee W et al (1989) Central hemodynamic assessment of normal term pregnancy. Am J Obstet Gynecol 161: 1439–1442.
9. Lucius H, Gahlenbeck H, Kleine H-O, Fabel H, Bartels H (1970) Respiratory functions, buffer system, and electrolyte concentrations of blood during human pregnancy. Resp Physiol 9: 311–317.
10. Gazioglu K, Kaltreider NL, Rosen M, Yu PN (1970) Pulmonary function during pregnancy in normal women and in patients with cardiopulmonary disease. Thorax 25: 445–450.
11. De Swiet M (1991) The respiratory system. In: Hytten F, Chamberlain G (eds) Clinical physiology in obstetrics, 2nd edn, pp. 83–100. Blackwell Scientific, Oxford.
12. Cuckle HS, Wald NJ, Thompson SG (1987) Estimating a woman's risk of having a pregnancy associated with Down's syndrome using her age and serum α-fetoprotein level. Br J Obstet Gynaecol 94: 387–402. Blackwell Science Ltd.
13. Ferguson-Smith M (1983) Prenatal chromosome analysis and its impact on the birth incidence of chromosome disorders. Br Med Bull 39: 355–364.
14. Robertson EG, Cheyne GA (1972) Plasma biochemistry in relation to the oedema of pregnancy. J Obstet Gynaecol Br Comm 79: 769–776. With permission, Blackwell Science Ltd.
15. Mendenhall HW (1970) Serum protein concentrations in pregnancy. Am J Obstet Gynecol 106: 388–399.
16. Adeniyi FA, Olatunbosun DA (1984) Origins and significance of the increased plasma alkaline phosphatase during normal pregnancy and pre-eclampsia. Br J Obstet Gynaecol 91: 857–862. Blackwell Science Ltd.
17. Girling JC, Dow E, Smith JH (1997) Liver function tests in pre-eclampsia: importance of comparison with a reference range derived for normal pregnancy. Br J Obstet Gynaecol 104: 246–250. Blackwell Science Ltd.
18. Heikkinene J, Mäentausta O, Ylöstalo P, Jänne O (1981) Changes in serum bile acid concentrations during normal pregnancy, in patients with intrahepatic cholestasis of pregnancy and in pregnant women with itching. Br J Obstet Gynaecol 88: 240–245. Blackwell Science Ltd.
19. Walker FB, Hoblit DL, Cunningham FG, Combes B (1974) Gamma glutamyl transpeptidase in normal pregnancy. Obstet Gynecol 43: 745–749.
20. McNair RD, Jaynes RV (1960) Alterations in liver function during normal pregnancy. Am J Obstet Gynecol 80: 500–505.
21. Kiiholma P, Gronroos M, Liukko P, Pakarinen P, Hyora H, Erkkola R (1984). Maternal serum copper and zinc concentrations in normal and small-for-date pregnancies. Gynecol Obstet Invest 18: 212–216.
22. Potter JM, Nestel PJ (1979) The hyperlipidaemia of pregnancy in normal and complicated pregnancies. Am J Obstet Gynecol 133: 165–170.
23. Lind T, Godfrey KA, Otun H (1984) Changes in serum uric acid concentrations during normal pregnancy. Br J Obstet Gynaecol 91: 128–132. Blackwell Science Ltd.
24. Newman RL (1957) Serum electrolytes in pregnancy, parturition, and puerperium. Obstet Gynecol 10: 51–55.

25. Kuhlback B, Widholm O (1966) Plasma creatinine in normal pregnancy. Scand J Clin Lab Invest 18: 654–656.
26. Davison J (1989) Renal disease. In: de Swiet M (ed) Medical disorders in obstetric practice, 2nd edn, pp. 306–407. Blackwell Scientific, Oxford.
27. Davison JM, Noble MCB (1981) Serial changes in 24 hour creatinine clearance during normal menstrual cycles and the first trimester of pregnancy. Br J Obstet Gynaecol 88: 10–17. With permission, Blackwell Science Ltd.
28. Davison JM, Dunlop W, Ezimokhai M (1980) 24-hour creatinine clearance during the third trimester of normal pregnancy. Br J Obstet Gynaecol 87: 106–109. Blackwell Science Ltd.
29. Davison JM, Dunlop W (1980) Renal haemodynamics and tubular function in normal human pregnancy. Kidney Int 18: 152–161.
30. Hytten FE, Cheyne GA (1972) The aminoaciduria of pregnancy. J Obstet Gynaecol Br Comm 79: 424–432.
31. Lopez-Espinola I, Dhar H, Humphreys S, Redman CWG (1986) Urinary albumin excretion in pregnancy. Br J Obstet Gynaecol 93: 176–181.
32. Lind T, Billewicz WZ, Brown G (1973) A serial study of changes occurring in the oral glucose tolerance test during pregnancy. J Obstet Gynaecol Br Comm 80: 1033–1039. Blackwell Science Ltd.
33. Mills JL, Jovanovic L, Knopp R et al (1998) Physiological reduction in fasting plasma glucose concentration in the first trimester of normal pregnancy: the diabetes in early pregnancy study. Metabolism 47: 1140–1144.
34. Hatem M, Anthony F, Hogston P, Rowe DJF, Dennis KJ (1988) Reference values for 75 g oral glucose tolerance test in pregnancy. Br Med J 296: 676–678.
35. O'Sullivan JB, Mahan CM (1964) Criteria for the oral glucose tolerance test in pregnancy. Diabetes 13: 278–285.
36. Dicknson JE, Palmer SM (1990) Gestational diabetes: pathophysiology and diagnosis. Seminars Perinatol 14: 2–11.
37. Roberts AB, Baker JR (1986) Serum fructosamine: a screening test for diabetes in pregnancy. Am J Obstet Gynecol 154: 1027–1030.
38. Feige A, Nossner U (1985) Das Verhalten des glykosylierten Haemoglobins (Hb-Al) in normaler und pathologischer Schwangerschaft. Z Geburtshilfe Perinatol 189: 13–16.
39. Ylinen K, Hekalir R, Teramo K (1981) Haemoglobin A_{1c} during pregnancy of insulin-dependent diabetic and healthy control. J Obstet Gynaecol 1: 223–228.
40. Falluca F, Sciullo E, Napoli A, Cardellini G, Maldonato A (1995) Amniotic fluid insulin and C-peptide levels in diabetic and nondiabetic women during early pregnancy. J Clin Endocrinol Metab 81: 137–139.
41. Falluca F, Gargiulo P, Troili F et al (1985) Amniotic fluid insulin, C peptide concentrations, and fetal morbidity in infants of diabetic mothers. Am J Obstet Gynecol 153: 534–540.
42. Carpenter MW, Canick JA, Star J, Carr SR, Burke ME, Shahinian K (1996) Fetal hyperinsulinism at 14–20 weeks and subsequent gestational diabetes. Obstet Gynecol 87: 89–93.
43. Wang Y, Walsh SW, Guo J, Zhang J (1991) Maternal levels of prostacyclin, thromboxane, vitamin E, and lipid peroxides throughout normal pregnancy. Am J Obstet Gynecol 165: 1690–1694.
44. Ortega RM, Quintas ME, Andres P, Martinez RM, Lopez-Sobaler AM (1998) Ascorbic acid levels in maternal milk: differences with respect to ascorbic acid status during the third trimester of pregnancy. Br J Nutr 79: 431–437.
45. Taylor DJ, Lind T (1979) Red cell mass during and after normal pregnancy. Br J Obstet Gynaecol 86: 364–370. Blackwell Science Ltd.
46. Efrati P, Presentey B, Margalith M, Rozenszajn L (1964) Leukocytes of normal pregnant women. Obstet Gynecol 23: 429–432.
47. Kuvin SF, Brecher G (1962) Differential neutrophil counts in pregnancy. N Engl J Med 266: 877–878.
48. Fay RA, Hughes AO, Farron NT (1983) Platelets in pregnancy: hyperdestruction in pregnancy. Obstet Gynecol 61: 238–240. The American College of Obstetrics and Gynecology.
49. Fenton V, Saunders K, Cavill I (1977) The platelet count in pregnancy. J Clin Pathol 30: 68–69.
50. Fenton V, Cavill I, Fisher J (1977) Iron stores in pregnancy. Br J Haematol 37: 145–149. Blackwell Science Ltd.
51. Ek J, Magnus M (1981) Plasma and red blood cell folate during normal pregnancies. Acta Obstet Gynecol Scand 60: 247–251. Munskgaard International Publishers Limited, Copenhagen, Denmark.
52. Chanarin I, Rothman D, Ward A, Perry J (1968) Folate status and requirement in pregnancy. Br Med J 2: 390–394.

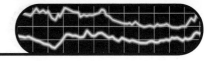

53. Walker MC, Smith GN, Perkins SL, Keely EJ, Garner PR (1999) Changes in homocysteine levels during normal pregnancy. Am J Obstet Gynecol 180: 660–664.
54. Letsky E (1991) The haematological system. In: Hytten F, Chamberlain G (eds) Clinical physiology in obstetrics, 2nd edn, pp. 39–82. Blackwell Scientific, Oxford.
55. Temperley IJ, Meehan MJM, Gatenby PBB (1968) Serum vitamin B12 levels in pregnant women. J Obstet Gynaecol Br Comm 75: 511–516. Blackwell Science Ltd.
56. Stirling Y, Woolf L, North WRS, Seghatchian MJ, Meade TW (1984) Haemostasis in normal pregnancy. Thromb Haemost 52: 176–182.
57. Warwick R, Hutton RA, Goff L, Letsky E, Heard M (1989) Changes in protein C and free protein S during pregnancy and following hysterectomy. J R Soc Med 82: 591–594.
58. Bonnar J, McNicol GP, Douglas AS (1969) Fibrinolytic enzyme system and pregnancy. Br Med J iii: 387–389.
59. Gallery ED, Raftos J, Gyory AZ, Wells JV (1981) A prospective study of serum complement (C3 and C4) levels during normal human pregnancy: effect of the development of pregnancy-associated hypertension. Aust NZ J Med 11: 243–245.
60. Schena FP, Manno C, Selvaggi L, Loverro G, Bettocchi S, Bonomo L (1982) Behaviour of immune complexes and the complement system in normal pregnancy and pre-eclampsia. J Clin Lab Immunol 7: 21–26.
61. Jenkins JS, Powell RJ (1987) C3 degradation products (C3d) in normal pregnancy. J Clin Pathol 40: 1362–1363.
62. Hytten FE, Lind T (1973) Volume and composition of the blood. In: Diagnostic indices in pregnancy, pp. 36–54. Documenta Geigy, Basle.
63. Haradaa, Hershman JM, Reed AW et al (1979) Comparison of thyroid stimulators and thyroid hormone concentrations in the sera of pregnant women. J Clin Endocrinol Metab 48: 793–797.
64. Man EB, Reid WA, Hellegers AE, Jones WS (1969) Thyroid function in human pregnancy. Am J Obstet Gynecol 103: 338–347.
65. Parker JH (1985) Amerlex free triiodothyronine and free thyroxine levels in normal pregnancy. Br J Obstet Gynaecol 92: 1234–1238. Blackwell Science Ltd.
66. Osathanondh R, Tulchinsky D, Chopra IJ (1976) Total and free thyroxine and triiodothyronine in normal and complicated pregnancy. J Clin Endocrinol Metab 42: 98–102.
67. Natrajan PG, McGarrigle HHG, Lawrence DM, Lachelin GCL (1982) Plasma noradrenaline and adrenaline levels in normal pregnancy and in pregnancy-induced hypertension. Br J Obstet Gynaecol 89: 1041–1045.
68. Rubin PC, Butters L, McCabe R, Reid JL (1986) Plasma catecholamines in pregnancy-induced hypertension. Clin Sci 71: 111–115.
69. Beilin LJ, Deacon J, Michael CA et al (1983) Diurnal rhythms of blood pressure, plasma renin activity, angiotensin II and catecholamines in normotensive and hypertensive pregnancies. Clin Exp Hypertension – Hypertension in Pregnancy B2(2): 271–293.
70. Carr BR, Parker CR, Madden JD, Macdonald PC, Porter JC (1981) Maternal plasma adrenocorticotrophin and cortisol relationships throughout human pregnancy. Am J Obstet Gynecol 139: 416–422.
71. Nolten WE, Lindheimer MD, Rueckert PA, Oparil S, Ehrlich EN (1980) Diurnal patterns and regulation of cortisol secretion in pregnancy. J Clin Endocrinol Metab 51: 466–472.
72. Rees LH, Burke CW, Chard T, Evans SW, Letchworth AT (1975) Possible placental origin of ACTH in normal human pregnancy. Nature 254: 620–622.
73. Doe RP, Fernandez R, Seal US (1964) Measurement of corticosteroid-binding globulin in man. J Clin Endocrinol 24: 1029–1039.
74. Migeon CJ, Kenny FM, Taylor FH (1968) Cortisol production rate VIII. Pregnancy. J Clin Endocrinol 28: 661–666.
75. Pearson Murphy BE, Okouneff LM, Klein GP, Ngo SH (1981) Lack of specificity of cortisol determinations in human urine. J Clin Endocrinol Metab 53: 91–99.
76. Nolten WE, Lindheimer MD, Oparil S, Ehrlich EN (1978) Desoxycorticosterone in normal pregnancy. I. Sequential studies of the secretory patterns of desoxycorticosterone, aldosterone, and cortisol. Am J Obstet Gynecol 132: 414–420.
77. Garner PR (1995) Pituitary and adrenal disorders. In: Burrow GN, Ferris TF (eds) Medical complications during pregnancy, 4th edn, pp. 188–209. WB Saunders, Philadelphia.
78. Biswas S, Rodek CH (1976) Plasma prolactin levels during pregnancy. Br J Obstet Gynaecol 83: 683–687. Blackwell Science Ltd.
79. Boyer RM, Finkelstein JW, Kapen S, Hellman L (1975) Twenty-four hour prolactin (Prl) secretory patterns during pregnancy. J Clin Endocrinol Metab 40: 1117–1120.

80. Rigg LA, Yen SSC (1977) Multiphasic prolactin secretion during parturition in human subjects. Am J Obstet Gynecol 128: 215–218.
81. Jacobs HS (1991) The hypothalamus and pituitary gland. In: Hytten F, Chamberlain G (eds) Clinical physiology in obstetrics, 2nd edn, pp. 345–356. Blackwell Scientific, Oxford.
82. Pitkin RM, Reynolds WA, Williams GA, Hargis GK (1979) Calcium metabolism in normal pregnancy: a longitudinal study. Am J Obstet Gynecol 133: 781–787.
83. Seki K, Makimura N, Mitsui C, Hirata J, Nagata I (1991) Calcium-regulating hormones and osteocalcin levels during pregnancy: a longitudinal study. Am J Obstet Gynecol 164: 1248–1252.
84. Wald NJ, George L, Smith D, Densem JW, Petterson K (1996) Serum screening for Down's syndrome between 8 and 14 weeks of pregnancy. Br J Obstet Gynaecol 103: 407–412. Blackwell Science Ltd.
85. Biagiotti R, Brizzi L, Periti E, D'Agata A, Vanzi E, Cariati E (1998) First trimester screening for Down's syndrome using maternal serum PAPP-A and free β-HCG in combination with fetal nuchal translucency thickness. Br J Obstet Gynaecol 105: 917–920.
86. Seppala M, Ruoslahti E (1972) Radioimmunoassay of maternal alpha fetoprotein during pregnancy and delivery. Am J Obstet Gynecol 112: 208–212.
87. Haddow JE, Palomaki GE (1992) Maternal protein enzyme analyses. In: Reece EA, Hobbins JC, Mahoney MJ, Petrie RH (eds) Medicine of the fetus and mother, pp. 653–667. JB Lippincott, Philadelphia.
88. Batzer FR, Schlaff S, Goldfarb AF, Corson SL (1981) Serial β-subunit human chorionic gonadotrophin doubling time as a prognosticator of pregnancy outcome in an infertile population. Fertil Steril 35: 307–311.
89. Brody S, Carlstrom G (1965) Human chorionic gonadotrophin pattern in serum and its relation to the sex of the fetus. J Clin Endocrinol 25: 792–797.
90. Josimovich JB, Kosor B, Boccella L, Mintz DH, Hutchinson DL (1970) Placental lactogen in maternal serum as an index of fetal health. Obstet Gynecol 36: 244–250. The American College of Obstetricians and Gynecologists.
91. Beck P, Parker ML, Daughaday WH (1965) Radioimmunologic measurement of human placental lactogen in plasma by a double antibody method during normal and diabetic pregnancies. J Clin Endocrinol 25: 1457–1462.
92. Mathur RS, Leaming AB, Williamson HO (1972) A simplified method for estimation of estriol in pregnancy plasma. Am J Obstet Gynecol 113: 1120–1129.
93. Mills MS (1992) Ultrasonography of early embryonic growth and fetal development. MD thesis, University of Bristol.
94. Robinson HP, Fleming JEE (1975) A critical evaluation of sonar 'crown–rump length' measurements. Br J Obstet Gynaecol 82: 702–710. Blackwell Science Ltd.
95. Pedersen JF (1982) Fetal crown–rump length measurement by ultrasound in normal pregnancy. Br J Obstet Gynaecol 89: 926–930.
96. Parker AJ, Davies P, Newton JR (1982) Assessment of gestational age of the Asian fetus by the sonar measurement of crown–rump length and biparietal diameter. Br J Obstet Gynaecol 89: 836–838.
97. Nicolaides KH, Azar G, Byrne D, Mansur C, Marks K (1992) Fetal nuchal translucency: ultrasound screening for chromosomal defects in first trimester of pregnancy. Br Med J 304: 867–869.
98. Pandya PP, Snijders RM, Johnson SP, Brizot ML, Nicolaides KH (1995) Screening for fetal trisomies by maternal age and fetal nuchal translucency thickness at 10–14 weeks of gestation. Br J Obstet Gynecol 102: 957–962. Blackwell Science Ltd.
99. Nicolaides KH, Brizot ML, Snijders RJM (1994) Fetal nuchal translucency: ultrasound screening for fetal trisomy in the first trimester of pregnancy. Br J Obstet Gynaecol 101: 782–786.
100. Altman DG, Chitty LS (1994) Charts of fetal size: 1. Methodology. Br J Obstet Gynecol 101: 29–34. Blackwell Science Ltd.
101. Chitty LS, Altman DG, Henderson A, Campbell S (1994) Charts of fetal size: 2. Head measurements. Br J Obstet Gynecol 101: 35–43. Blackwell Science Ltd.
102. Kurmanavicius J, Wright EM, Royston P, Wisser J, Huch R, Huch A, Zimmermann R (1999) Fetal ultrasound biometry: 1. Head reference values. Br J Obstet Gynaecol 106: 126–135.
103. Snijders RJM, Nicolaides KH (1994) Fetal biometry at 14–40 weeks' gestation. Ultrasound Obstet Gynecol 4: 34–48. Blackwell Science Limited.
104. Erikson PS, Secher NJ, Weis-Bentzon M (1985) Normal growth of the fetal biparietal diameter and the abdominal diameter in a longitudinal study. Acta Obstet Gynecol Scand 64: 65–70.
105. Hadlock FP, Deter RL, Harrist RB, Park SK (1982) Fetal head circumference: relation to menstrual age. Am J Roentgenol 138: 647–653.

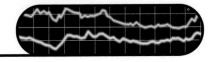

106. Chitty LS, Altman DG, Henderson A, Campbell S (1994). Charts of fetal size: 3. Abdominal measurements. Br J Obstet Gynecol 101: 125–131.
107. Kurmanavicius J, Wright EM, Royston P et al (1999) Fetal ultrasound biometry: 2. Abdomen and femur length reference values. Br J Obstet Gynaecol 106: 136–143.
108. Hadlock FP, Deter RL, Harrist RB, Park SK (1982) Fetal abdominal circumference as a predictor of menstrual age. Am J Roentgenol 139: 367–370.
109. Deter RL, Harrist RB, Hadlock FP, Poindexteran (1982) Longitudinal studies of fetal growth with the use of dynamic image ultrasonography. Am J Obstet Gynecol 143: 545–554.
110. Tamura RK, Sabbagha RE (1980) Percentile ranks for sonar fetal abdominal circumference measurements. Am J Obstet Gynecol 138: 475–479.
111. Chitty LS, Altman DG, Henderson A, Campbell S (1994) Charts of fetal size: 4. Femur length. Br J Obstet Gynecol 101: 132–135. Blackwell Science Ltd.
112. Warda AH, Deter RL, Rossavik IK, Carpenter RJ, Hadlock FP (1985) Fetal femur length: a critical reevaluation of the relationship to menstrual age. Obstet Gynecol 66: 69–75.
113. Chitty LS, Altman DG (1993) Charts of fetal size. In: Dewbury K, Meire H, Cosgrove D (eds) Ultrasound in obstetrics and gynaecology, pp. 513–595. Churchill Livingstone, Edinburgh.
114. Merz E, Kim-Kern M-S, Pehl S (1987) Ultrasonic mensuration of fetal limb bones in the second and third trimesters. J Clin Ultrasound 15: 175–183.
115. Jeanty P (1991) Fetal biometry. In: Fleischer AC, Romero R, Manning FA, Jeanty P, James AE (eds) The principles and practice of ultrasonography in obstetrics and gynecology, 4th edn, pp. 93–108. Appleton and Lange, Norwalk, CT.
116. Romero R, Athanassiadis AP, Sirtori M, Inati M (1991) Fetal skeletal anomalies. In: Fleischer AC, Romero R, Manning FA, Jeanty P, James AE (eds) The principles and practice of ultrasonography in obstetrics and gynecology, 4th edn, pp. 277–306. Appleton and Lange, Norwalk, CT.
117. Grannum P, Bracken M, Silverman R, Hobbins JC (1980) Assessment of fetal kidney size in normal gestation by comparison of ratio of kidney circumference to abdominal circumference. Am J Obstet Gynecol 136: 249–254.
118. Mayden KL, Tortora M, Berkowitz RL, Bracken M, Hobbins JC (1982) Orbital diameters: a new parameter for prenatal diagnosis and dating. Am J Obstet Gynecol 144: 289–297.
119. Goldstein I, Reece EA, Pilu G, Bovicelli L, Hobbins JC (1987) Cerebellar measurements with ultrasonography in the evaluation of fetal growth and development. Am J Obstet Gynecol 156: 1065–1069.
120. Roberts AB, Mitchell JM, Pattison NS (1989). Fetal liver length in normal and isoimmunised pregnancies. Am J Obstet Gynecol 161: 42–46.
121. Shimizu T, Salvador L, Allanson J, Hughes-Benzie R, Nimrod C (1992) Ultrasonographic measurements of fetal ear. Obstet Gynecol 80: 381–384.
122. Birnholz JC, Farrell E (1988) Fetal ear length. Pediatrics 81: 555–558.
123. Reece EA, Yarkoni S, Abdalla M et al (1991) A prospective longitudinal study of growth in twin gestations compared with growth in singleton pregnancies. I. The fetal head. J Ultrasound Med 10: 439–443.
124. Reece EA, Yarkoni S, Abdalla M et al (1991) A prospective longitudinal study of growth in twin gestations compared with growth in singleton pregnancies. II. The fetal limbs. J Ultrasound Med 10: 445–450.
125. Socol ML, Tamura RK, Sabbagha RE, Chen T, Vaisrub N (1984) Diminished biparietal diameter and abdominal circumference growth in twins. Obstet Gynecol 64: 235–238.
126. Grumbach K, Coleman BG, Arger PH, Mintz MC, Gabbe SV, Mennuti MT (1986) Twin and singleton growth patterns compared using US. Radiology 158: 237–241.
127. Shushan A, Mordel N, Zajicek G, Lewin A, Schenker JG, Sadovsky E (1993) A comparison of sonographic growth curves of triplet and twin fetuses. Am J Perinatol 10: 388–391.
128. Wilcox M, Gardosi J, Mongelli M, Ray C, Johnson I (1993) Birth weight from pregnancies dated by ultrasonography in a multicultural British population. Br Med J 307: 588–591.
129. Yudkin PL, Aboualfa M, Eyre JA, Redman CWG, Wilkinson AR (1987) New birthweight and head circumference centiles for gestational ages 24 to 42 weeks. Early Hum Dev 15: 45–52.
130. Thompson AM, Billewicz WZ, Hytten FE (1968) The assessment of fetal growth. J Obstet Gynaecol Br Comm 75: 903–916.
131. Wilcox MA, Johnson IR, Maynard PV, Smith SJ, Chilvers CED (1993) The individualised birthweight ratio: a more logical outcome measure of pregnancy than birthweight alone. Br J Obstet Gynaecol 100: 342–347.
132. Williams RL, Creasy RK, Cunningham GC, Hawes WE, Norris FD, Tashiro M (1982) Fetal growth and perinatal viability in California. Obstet Gynecol 59: 624–632.

133. Campbell S, Wilkin D (1975) Ultrasonic measurement of fetal abdomen circumference in the estimation of fetal weight. Br J Obstet Gynaecol 82: 689–697. Blackwell Science Ltd.
134. Shepard MJ, Richards VA, Berkowitz RL, Warsof SL, Hobbins JC (1982) An evaluation of two equations for predicting fetal weight by ultrasound. Am J Obstet Gynecol 142: 47–54.
135. Hadlock FP, Harrist RB, Carpenter RJ, Deter RL, Park SK (1984) Sonographic estimation of fetal weight. Radiology 150: 535–540.
136. Brace RA, Wolf EJ (1989) Normal amniotic fluid volume changes throughout pregnancy. Am J Obstet Gynecol 161: 382–388.
137. Moore TR, Cayle JE (1990) The amniotic fluid index in normal human pregnancy. Am J Obstet Gynecol 162: 1168–1173.
138. Fisk NM, Ronderos-Dumit D, Tannirandorn Y, Nicolini U, Talbert D (1992) Normal amniotic pressure throughout gestation. Br J Obstet Gynaecol 99: 18–22. Blackwell Science Ltd.
139. Gilbert WM, Moore TR, Brace RA (1991) Amniotic fluid volume dynamics. Fetal Med Rev 3: 89–104. Cambridge University Press.
140. Lind T, Parkin FM, Cheyne GA (1969) Biochemical and cytological changes in liquor amnii with advancing gestation. J Obstet Gynaecol Br Comm 76: 673–683.
141. Saddiqi TA, Meyer RA, Korfhagen J, Khoury JC, Rosenn B, Miodovnik M (1993) A longitudinal study describing confidence limits of normal fetal cardiac, thoracic and pulmonary dimensions from 20 to 40 weeks gestation. J Ultrasound Med 12: 731–736.
142. Steed RD, Strickland DM, Swanson MS et al (1998) Normal fetal cardiac dimensions obtained by perpendicular imaging. Am J Cardiol 81: 1059–1061. Excerpta Medica Inc.
143. Tan J, Silverman NH, Hoffman JIE, Villegas M, Schmidt KG (1992) Cardiac dimensions determined by cross-sectional echocardiography in the normal human fetus from 18 weeks to term. Am J Cardiol 70: 1459–1467. Excerpta Medica Inc.
144. Rizzo G, Capponi A, Arduini D, Romanini C (1994) Ductus venosus velocity waveforms in appropriate and small for gestational age fetuses. Early Hum Dev 39: 15–26. Elsevier Science.
145. Hecher K, Campbell S, Snijders R, Nicolaides K (1994) Reference ranges for fetal venous and atrioventricular blood flow parameters. Ultrasound Obstet Gynecol 4: 381–390. Blackwell Science Limited.
146. Rizzo G, Arduini D, Romanini C (1992) Inferior vena cava flow velocity waveforms in appropriate- and small-for-gestational-age fetuses. Am J Obstet Gynecol 166: 1271–1280.
147. Rizzo G, Capponi A, Talone PE, Arduini D, Romanini C (1996) Doppler indices from inferior vena cava and ductus venosus in predicting pH and oxygen tension in umbilical blood at cordocentesis in growth-retarded fetuses. Ultrasound Obstet Gynecol 7: 401–410.
148. Hecher K, Snijders R, Campbell S, Nicolaides K (1995) Fetal venous, intracardiac, and arterial blood flow measurements in intrauterine growth retardation: Relationship with fetal blood gases. Am J Obstet Gynecol 173: 10–15.
149. Rizzo G, Arduini D (1991) Fetal cardiac function in intrauterine growth retardation. Am J Obstet Gynecol 165: 876–882.
150. Van Splunder P, Stijnen T, Wladimiroff JW (1997) Fetal atrioventricular, venous and arterial flow velocity waveforms in the small for gestational age fetus. Pediatr Res 42: 765–775.
151. Mari G, Deter RL, Uerpairojkit B (1996) Flow velocity waveforms of the ductus arteriosus in appropriate and small-for-gestational age fetuses. J Clin Ultrasound 24: 185–196.
152. Rizzo G, Capponi A, Chaoui R, Taddei F, Arduini D, Romanini C (1996) Blood flow velocity waveforms from peripheral pulmonary arteries in normally grown and growth-retarded fetuses. Ultrasound Obstet Gynecol 8: 87–92.
153. Arduini D, Rizzo G (1990) Normal values of Pulsatility Index from fetal vessels: A cross-sectional study on 1556 healthy fetuses. J Perinat Med 18: 165–172.
154. Mari G, Adrignolo A, Abuhamad AZ et al (1995) Diagnosis of fetal anemia with Doppler ultrasound in the pregnancy complicated by maternal blood group immunisation. Ultrasound Obstet Gynecol 5: 400–405. Blackwell Science Limited.
155. Mari G, Deter RL (1992) Middle cerebral artery flow velocity waveforms in normal and small-for-gestational-age fetuses. Am J Obstet Gynecol 166: 1262–1270.
156. Veille J-C, Hanson R, Tatum K (1993) Longitudinal quantitation of middle cerebral artery blood flow in normal human fetuses. Am J Obstet Gynecol 169: 1393–1398.
157. Kurmanavicius J, Florio I, Wisser J et al. (1997) Reference resistance indices of the umbilical, fetal middle cerebral and uterine arteries at 24–42 weeks of gestation. Ultrasound Obstet Gynecol 10: 112–120. Blackwell Science Limited.
158. Vyas S, Nicolaides KH, Bower S, Campbell S (1990) Middle cerebral artery flow velocity waveforms in fetal hypoxaemia. Br J Obstet Gynaecol 97: 797–803.

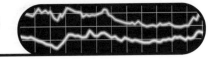

159. Sherer DM (1997) Prenatal ultrasonographic assessment of the middle cerebral artery: A review. Obstet Gynecol Survey 52: 444–455.

160. Erskine RLA, Ritchie JWK (1985) Umbilical artery blood flow characteristics in normal and growth-retarded fetuses. Br J Obstet Gynaecol 92: 605–610. Blackwell Science Limited.

161. Bahado-Singh RO, Kovanci E, Jeffres A et al (1999) The Doppler cerebroplacental ratio and perinatal outcome in intrauterine growth restriction. Am J Obstet Gynecol 180: 750–756.

162. Weiner CP, Sipes SL, Wenstrom K (1992) The effect of fetal age upon normal fetal laboratory values and venous pressure. Obstet Gynecol 79: 713–718.

163. Weiner CP, Heilskov J, Pelzer G, Grant S, Wenstrom K, Williamson RA (1989) Normal values for human umbilical venous and amniotic fluid pressures and their alteration by fetal disease. Am J Obstet Gynecol 161: 714–717.

164. Weiner CP (1995) Intrauterine pressure: amniotic and fetal circulation. In: Ludomirski A, Nicolini U, Bhutani UK (eds) Therapeutic and diagnostic interventions in early life, ch 4. Futura, New York.

165. Sadovsky G, Nicolaides KH (1989) Reference ranges for fetal heart rate patterns in normoxaemic nonanaemic fetuses. Fetal Ther 4: 61–68.

166. Arulkumaran S, Ingemarsson I, Montan S et al (1992) Guidelines for interpretation of antepartum and intrapartum cardiotocography. Hewlett Packard, Bracknell.

167. NIH Workshop (1997) Electronic fetal heart rate monitoring: research guidelines for interpretation. Am J Obstet Gynecol 177: 1385–1390.

168. Manning FA, Platt LD, Sipos L (1980) Antepartum fetal evaluation: Development of a fetal biophysical profile. Am J Obstet Gynecol 136: 787–795.

169. Manning FA, Baskett TF, Morrison I, Lange I (1981) Fetal biophysical profile scoring: A prospective study in 1184 high-risk patients. Am J Obstet Gynecol 140: 289–294.

170. Takagi K, Tanaka H, Nishijima S et al (1989) Fetal blood values by percutaneous umbilical blood sampling. Fetal Diagnosis & Therapy 4: 152–160.

171. Forestier F (1987) Some aspects of fetal biology. Fetal Ther 2: 181–187.

172. Weiner CP (1992) Human fetal bilirubin levels and fetal hemolytic disease. Am J Obstet Gynecol 166: 1449–1454.

173. Economides DL, Nicolaides KH, Campbell S (1991) Metabolic and endocrine findings in appropriate and small for gestational age fetuses. J Perinat Med 19: 97–105.

174. Nicolini U, Fisk NM, Rodeck CH, Beacham J (1992) Fetal urine biochemistry: an index of renal maturation and dysfunction. Br J Obstet Gynaecol 99: 46–50. Blackwell Science Ltd.

175. Nicolaides KH, Cheng HH, Snijders RJM, Moniz CF (1992) Fetal urine biochemistry in the assessment of obstructive uropathy. Am J Obstet Gynecol 166: 932–937.

176. Evans MI, Sacks AJ, Johnson MP, Robichaux AG, May M, Moghissi KS (1991) Sequential invasive assessment of fetal renal function and the intrauterine treatment of fetal obstructive uropathies. Obstet Gynecol 77: 545–550.

177. Wilkins IA, Chitkara U, Lynch L, Goldberg JD, Mehalek KE, Berkowitz RL (1987) The nonpredictive value of fetal urinary electrolytes: preliminary report of outcomes and correlations with pathological diagnosis. Am J Obstet Gynecol 157: 694–698.

178. Huch A, Huch R, Rooth G (1994) Guidelines for blood sampling and measurement of pH and blood gas values in obstetrics. Eur J Obstet Gynaecol Reprod Biol 54: 165–175. Elsevier Science.

179. Nicolaides KH, Economides DL, Soothill PW (1989) Blood gases, pH, and lactate in appropriate- and small-for-gestational-age fetuses. Am J Obstet Gynecol 161: 996–1001.

180. Soothill PW, Nicolaides KH, Rodeck CH, Campbell S (1986) Effect of gestational age on fetal and intervillous blood gas and acid–base values in human pregnancy. Fetal Ther 1: 168–175.

181. Nicolaides KH, Thilaganathan B, Mibashan RS (1989) Cordocentesis in the investigation of fetal erythropoiesis. Am J Obstet Gynecol 161: 1197–1200.

182. Weiner CP, Williamson RA, Wenstrom KD, Sipes SL, Grant SS, Widness JA (1991) Management of fetal hemolytic disease by cordocentesis. I. Prediction of fetal anemia. Am J Obstet Gynecol 165: 546–553.

183. Davies NP, Buggins AGS, Snijders RJM, Jenkins E, Layton DM, Nicolaides KH (1992) Blood leucocyte count in the human fetus. Arch Dis Child 67: 399–403.

184. Abbas A, Thilaganathan B, Buggins AGS, Layton DM, Nicolaides KH (1993) Fetal plasma interferon gamma concentration in normal pregnancy. Am J Obstet Gynecol 168: 1414–1416.

185. Weiner CP (1995) Unpublished data.

186. Nicolaides KH, Rodeck CH, Mibashan RS, Kemp JR (1986) Have Liley charts outlived their usefulness? Am J Obstet Gynecol 155: 90–94.

187. Thorpe-Beeston JG, Nicolaides KH, Felton CV, Butler J, McGregor AM (1991) Maturation of the secretion of thyroid hormone and thyroid stimulating hormone in the fetus. N Engl J Med

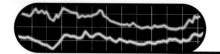
324: 532–536. With permission, Massachussetts Medical Society.

188. Duignan NM, Studd JWW, Hughes AO (1975) Characteristics of normal labour in different racial groups. Br J Obstet Gynaecol 82: 593–601. Blackwell Science Ltd.

189. Eskes TKAB, Jongsma HW, Houx PCW (1983) Percentiles for gas values in human umbilical cord blood. Europ J Obstet Gynec Reprod Biol 14: 341–346. Elsevier Science.

190. Westgren M, Divon M, Horal M et al (1995) Routine measurements of umbilical artery lactate levels in the prediction of perinatal outcome. Am J Obstet Gynecol 173: 1416–1422.

191. Mercelina-Roumans P, Breukers R, Ubachs J, Van Wersch J (1996) Hematological variables in cord blood of neonates of smoking and nonsmoking mothers. J Clin Epidemiol 49: 449–454. Elsevier Science.

192. Paterakis GS, Lykopoulou L, Papassotiriou J, Stamulakatou A, Kattamis C, Loukopoulos D (1993) Flow-cytometric analysis of reticulocytes in normal cord blood. Acta Haematol 90: 182–185.

193. Walka MM, Sonntag J, Kage A, Dudenhausen JW, Obladen M (1998) Complete blood counts from umbilical cords of healthy term newborns by two automated cytometers. Acta Haematol 100: 167–173.

194. Perkins SL, Livesey JF, Belcher J (1993) Reference intervals for 21 clinical chemistry analytes in arterial and venous cord blood. Clin Chem 39: 1041–1044.

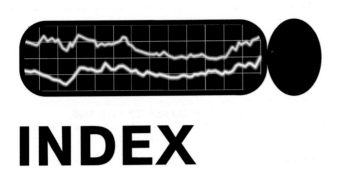

INDEX

INDEX

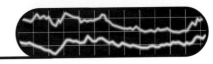

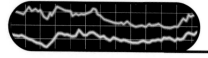

INDEX

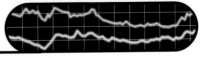

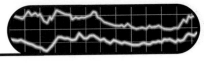

INDEX